# LEARNING TO CARE in the OPERATING DEPARTMENT

# LEARNING TO CARE IN THE OPERATING DEPARTMENT

**Kate Nightingale** RGN, RMN, RCNT Cert. Ed
Lecturer, Norfolk College of Nursing, Norfolk, UK

**Doreen Kalideen** BEd (Hons), RGN, RCNT Cert. Ed (FE), DipN (Lond)
Lecturer, Nightingale Institute, London, UK

**Margaret Heaton** RGN, RNT Cert Ed, RCNT, BSc (Hons) Nursing Studies
Lecturer, West Yorkshire College of Health Studies, Wakefield, UK

Edward Arnold
A member of the Hodder Headline Group
LONDON MELBOURNE AUCKLAND

First published in Great Britain 1987
Second edition 1995

*British Library Cataloguing in Publication Data*
A catalogue record for this book is available from the British Library

ISBN 0 340 59492 6



Typeset in 10/11 pt Times by J&L Composition Ltd, Filey, North Yorkshire
Printed and bound in Great Britain for Edward Arnold, a division of Hodder Headline, 338 Euston Road, London NW1 3BH by
J.W. Arrowsmith Ltd, Bristol

# Contents

# Acknowledgements

The authors wish to thank Wendy Ellis and Anita Burke for their permission to use the care studies on which Chapter 9 is based.

Mrs. Oakley's care study was completed by Wendy during a post-registration Critical Care course in the Norfolk College of Nursing, Norwich and Mr. Smith's care study was undertaken by Anita whilst she was a student on the ENB course at the Nightingale and Guy's College of Health, St. Thomas' Hospital, London.

The names of the patients have been changed to protect their identity.

# Preface

This is the second edition of *Learning to Care in the Operating Department*. It is difficult to grasp how much has changed in the few years since the first edition was published. The health services have gone through a major reorganisation; nursing and nurse education have changed and, at the same time, a major revolution in surgical techniques has taken place. As a result three of the contributors to the first edition have come together to rewrite the contents for a new generation of nursing students.

The experience of the operating department may be very brief for some students, perhaps whilst based in a surgical ward and following a patient through their peri-operative progress. Others may be allocated to the operating department for a short time or may wish to observe a surgical anaesthetic procedure.

At the same time there are other students in the department, operating department practitioners or nurses who have chosen to practise in this speciality. For everyone there is always that first time, when one is new to the operating department and to caring for patients at a time of great stress.

The purpose of this book is to stimulate the student to find answers to some of the questions they will be asking in an environment which is rapidly changing at the best of times. The book is patient centred and student focused. It is not concerned with the development of the technical skills of the operating department. It is about nursing care during the peri-operative period. Whilst giving some insights into policies and protocols, it attempts to encourage the student to reflect on his or her contribution to the successful care of the patient during the peri-operative period.

The academic level has been readjusted to meet the needs of the present day nursing student but it is structured so that it can be used by a variety of students. Some may wish to explore peri-operative care in more depth. Others may only gain a brief insight into what goes on in the theatre. This book will, we hope, help you to make the most of your experience in this very different environment, provide you with some principles for practice and help you to focus on how patient needs are met during this vulnerable time.

# Introduction

In recent years there have been enormous changes in health care. The curriculum for preregistration nurse education has also changed.[1] We have joined the European Community. We have become increasingly aware of environmental threats to both ourselves and to the environment itself.

There has also been a revolution in surgery due to the application of new technology to surgical practice: **minimally invasive surgery**, laser surgery, as well as the expected advances as new technology is applied to more conventional surgery, not to mention new anaesthetic agents which promote early patient recovery with minimal side effects and day surgery. By the year 2000 it is anticipated that more than 50% of surgery will be carried out as day procedures.[2] Although pre-registration nursing students in some colleges are no longer placed in the **operating department**, this is not universal and there will be students who will wish to spend some time in the department on an elective basis.

Increasing awareness of environmental hazards and of the rise in the incidence of bloodborne viral infections have also had their effect. Theatre practices have changed to incorporate new regulations which are now clearly defined and monitored by both national and international agencies, ranging from the World Health Organisation through European directives to the Health and Safety Executive.[3,4] Guidelines for practice are also maintained by professional organisations, such as the National Association of Theatre Nurses.[5,6,7,8,9]

Although this book is still aimed at the preregistration student nurse the authors are aware that new members of the theatre team may also find it useful as the book addresses issues of peri-operative patient care which are often obscured by the more technical aspects of operating department work. **Operating Department Practitioners** (ODPs) may have some experience in the department before starting a National Vocational Qualification (**NVQ**) course but, equally, they may not. They will certainly have little understanding of how nurses assess, plan and evaluate the care they give to meet individual needs of patients.

The authors have also borne in mind the fact that the first edition of this book was used by theatre staff who were then only beginning to apply the principles of peri-operative nursing to practice. It is hoped that this edition will be of some use in carrying forward the development of the independent nursing role of those nurses who work in a truly interdisciplinary theatre team as well as enabling the preregistration student to develop an understanding of the peri-operative role of the nurse.

The style of the book has been changed. Activities in the text are designed to guide the student in achieving key learning outcomes and are intended to be completed under the supervision of a nurse who is in a **mentor** or preceptor relationship with the student.

The following are standard operating department texts which should be available in any operating department or in the library of a school of nursing.

Atkinson RS *et al.* (1993) *Synopsis of Anaesthesia*, 11th edn. Butterworth Heinemann, London.
Brigden RJ (1988) *Operating Theatre Technique*, 5th edn. Churchill Livingstone, Edinburgh.
Drain C and Christoph SS (1987) *The Recovery Room: A Critical Care Approach to Post Anaesthesia Nursing*. WB Saunders, Philadelphia.
Kneedler JS and Dodge GH (1987) *Perioperative Patient Care. The Nursing Perspective*, 3rd edn. Blackwell, Boston.
Meeker MH and Rothrock J (1991) *Alexander's Care of the Patient in Surgery*, 19th edn. Mosby, St. Louis.
Rothrock J (1990) *Perioperative Nursing Care Planning*. Mosby, St. Louis.
West BM (1992) *Theatre Nursing Technique and Care*. Ballière, London.

The following journals have been referenced a number of times in the book and should be available in any nursing library running a course for nurses working in the operating department.

*American Operating Room Nurses Journal*
*British Journal of Theatre Nursing*

## References

1. Statutory instrument No. 1455. Nurses, Midwives and Health Visitors (Parts of the Register) Amendments (No.2) Order. (1989) HMSO, London.
2. NHS Management Executive (1993) *Report by Day Surgery Task Force*. HMSO, London.
3. Pediani, R (1993) Hazards and safety in theatre. *B J Theatre Nursing*, **2**(12), 19–21.

4. Health & Safety Executive (1992) *Workplace Health, Safety and Welfare Regulations. Approved Code of Practice.* HSE, Sheffield.
5. National Association of Theatre Nurses (1988) *Principles of Safe Practice in the Operating Theatre.* NATN, Harrogate.
6. Ibid. (1991) *A Strategy for Nursing in the Operating Department.*
7. Ibid. (1992) *The Named Nurse in the Operating Department.*
8. Ibid. (1993) *The Nurse as First Assistant.*
9. Medical Defence Union/RCN/NATN (1986) *Theatre Safeguards.* MDU/RCN/NATN, London.

# 1 Nursing in the Operating Theatre

'I never realised that patients needed so much nursing care when they went to theatres.'

This remark was made by a student during the evaluation of his four week placement in the operating department, when several of a group of students completed total patient care assessments.

It was an interesting insight. Without awareness of that part of the patient's experience which takes place between leaving the ward and returning several hours later, how can nurses expect to understand and meet the needs of their patients? During most operative or anaesthetic procedures the patient, even if not critically ill, will be highly dependent on the care and skills of the operating department team. There is a tendency to think only of the more technological aspects of treatment when thinking about **operative procedures**.

The patient undergoing surgery is still a person, with the very real needs, fears and problems of any other person, facing what is often a major life event. For the patient arriving for surgery there is the problem of passing through the care of many different groups of nurses. The medical staff do not change. The same group of doctors normally care for the patient on the ward and carry out the operation. There can be up to six groups of nurses, all with specialist skills, involved in the care of the patient between the time the patient is admitted for surgery and the time he returns to the ward, having recovered from the immediate effects of the operation.

The nurse's role as patient's **advocate** is extremely important during this time which we refer to as the **peri-operative period**.[1] The patient, normally, has very little knowledge of any of the procedures which are to take place in a strange and highly technical environment where people hide their faces behind masks. Because of their physical condition and because of what will be done during the operation, patients will not have the physical capabilities to look after their own safety. The patient may or may not be rendered unconscious by the administration of a **general anaesthetic**. If awake and receiving an operation under local **analgesia**, each patient is still dependent on those caring for them, possibly very sleepy due to the medication which will almost certainly have been given to relieve anxiety.

Nowadays, we would expect the patients to have been given sufficient information to allow them to give informed **consent** to the operation about to be undertaken.[2] Understanding what is about to happen has been shown to be valuable in relieving the anxiety inherent in facing a dangerous situation alone, in a strange environment and without the support we expect to have to cope in life.[3,4]

## Peri-operative care planning

The peri-operative period is not a fixed time. In a day care unit the peri-operative time may start as soon as the patient is referred from the outpatient appointment and the nurse from the day care unit visits to begin the pre-operative assessment. For traumatised patients, admitted through the Accident and Emergency Department (A&E), the peri-operative time may not start until the patient is in the anaesthetic room.

This raises the vexed question of documenting care for a patient during the peri-operative period. Writing care plans for surgical patients was ever difficult. Even the ward care plan changes rapidly over a period of 24 hours and many nursing models seem to have been designed for longer term and more slowly moving situations than this. How much more difficult, then, to write a care plan to include all the possible variables in the time immediately surrounding the actual operation. Some ward nurses would say that there is no need for a care plan for the time spent in the operating room whilst some people say that there is no need for a nurse in the operating department. The quotation at the head of this chapter should be sufficient justification.

Some nurses would say that the ward care plan will suffice. Most theatre nurses would disagree with this but will also point out that if you are carrying out care without having the opportunity to carry out a detailed assessment then you need a 'care record', not a care plan. Nurses in the operating department try to carry out pre-operative visits to meet their patient and assess their individual needs for care during the peri-operative period. Many have developed separate 'theatre care plans' which may or may not be an integral part of the overall care plan begun in the ward.[5]

One problem for theatre or recovery ward nurses has been how to organise their time to carry out pre-operative assessments by visiting their patients on the ward. This has been solved in different ways in different places. It has sometimes resulted in the drawing up of nursing documents which look more like check lists than detailed care plans. This reflects some of the issues which impinge on the peri-operative situation. If a comprehensive care plan accompanies the patient from the ward, the operating department nurses are working as part of a multidisciplinary team and should contribute to those documents rather than adding to the proliferation of paper work, all saying the same things in slightly different ways.

Operating departments are in the process of introducing computerised records. The anaesthetists like to have their own records and now there are management initiatives for computerised and comprehensive patient records. Whatever the situation, the ideal has often been compromised by the reality of practice.[6]

This book is patient centred. It will look at the patient not from the theatre staff viewpoint, not from the ward nurses' viewpoint, but from the viewpoint of the new student in the operating department. This means that we shall be giving you guidance to follow patients through and help you to use existing care plan tools in your own theatres or to devise your own to carry out a care study. It will also enable you to evaluate the effectiveness of both the tools and the care. But before you can do this you must have some introduction to a department which is not only strange to the patient but may also be strange to you. To function safely in a new and strange environment you need to feel reasonably comfortable that you are observing the rules, formal or informal. Operating departments, with their specialised procedures, clothes, barriers and changing rooms, can be a bit daunting in this respect. The next two chapters will provide a broad overview of basic operating theatre practice and uncover some of the mystique of 'theatre techniques'.

## *Activities*

Once you are established and have made contact with your clinical supervisor you may wish to complete the following questions. They can be answered after you have accompanied a patient to theatre whilst based on a ward or if you have been allowed to follow a patient through at an early stage of your placement.

If you are only spending a day or so in the department as part of your surgical placement, this activity may be as much as you can expect to complete.

1. Was a care plan written for your patient? How detailed was it? If not, how did the theatre team identify and meet the individual needs of the patient?
2. Who was the patient's named nurse? Is there a copy of *The Named Nurse in the Operating Department* in the theatre, or theatre department?

3. Which groups of nurses were involved in the care of the patient from leaving the ward to returning to ward?

4. Which of the following best describes the care your patient received?

   a) The patient was cared for safely.
   b) The patient was cared for safely and he/she felt comfortable and well supported.
   c) The patient was seen pre-operatively by a nurse from the operating department who helped to relieve the patient's anxiety, identified special needs and ensured the delivery of safe and effective nursing care throughout the peri-operative period.
   d) The operation was carried out safely and the theatre staff assisted the surgeon competently.

Discuss this with your clinical supervisor with special reference to the role of the nurse in the operating department.

5. Did you get a chance to study the operating department care plans and patient records? Did the realities of the working situation compromise the quality of the paper work and/or the implementation of the planned care?

## References

1. Webb, C (1987) Speaking up for advocacy. *N. Times*, **83**(34), 33–36.
2. Reid, J (1992) Informed consent. An ethical dilemma. *B J Theatre Nursing*, **2**(9), 23–25.
3. Boore, J (1988) Pre-operative information and post-operative recovery. *NatNews*, January, 16–22.
4. Hayward, J (1975) *Information: A Prescription Against Pain.* RCN, London.
5. Rothrock, J (1992) *Perioperative Care Planning*. C.V. Mosby, St. Louis.
6. Nightingale, K (1988) The ideal and the actual – pre-operative visiting re-visited. *NatNews*, **25**(12), 12.

# 2 Entering the Operating Theatre

It is always possible that the first day that you enter an unfamiliar theatre, a litle apprehensive that you have to change into strange clothes and walk, self-consciously, into this strange new place, could be the very day that every theatre in the department is working flat out. Two surgeons have started operating early ,a major and unusual operation is being carried out in one theatre, an emergency has just been admitted from A&E and síx members of staff, including your clinical supervisor, are off sick with stress related illnesses!

Yes, it can happen so it is as well to be prepared. There are two vital things to do. First, introduce yourself to your clinical supervisor in advance. This way you will be expected and someone will have been named to meet you and look after you during your first (or only) day in the department. You may have drafted objectives for a learning contract and this pre-visit will be your opportunity to start negotiations for an action plan which will enable you to achieve your objectives. It is important to define these objectives carefully in discussion with your own tutor or the specialist tutor for theatres.

It may be that there is no work pressure on your first day and your supervisor will have all the time in the world but, even so, it will be extremely helpful to you if you already have an understanding of the principles underlying safe practice in the operating theatre.[1] There are some very basic details of theatre practice with which the staff are so familiar that they may just tell you what to do rather than going into the basic principles of infection control or Health and Safety which underlie the practices.

### *Activity*

You might find it useful to regard this first introduction to theatres as a learning experience. Reflect on this and identify how your feelings can give you insights into how it feels to be a patient coming to theatre for surgery.

## Entering the operating theatre

In these days of high security it is sometimes impossible to get into an operating department without knowing the number for the security lock so you will have to report to the receptionist to be let into the changing rooms. Whether or not there is a security lock, do report to the receptionist and ask for the person who is to be your mentor for the day, as arranged at your pre-visit.

Your supervisor, or mentor, will take you into the changing room, show you a locker for your clothes and find a pair of shoes and theatre clothes for you. Try not to take valuables or more money than you need with you. Like all unattended places, theatre changing rooms are ready targets for opportunist thieves. Always lock away any money you have with you and the jewellery which you will be asked to remove before going into theatres. It is not a good idea to put jewellery in your theatre dress pocket. Many a watch or engagement ring has ended up in the laundry that way.

Donning theatre clothes is something of an art in itself if it is to be done safely. Some of the activities have become a bit of a ritual but there are well researched principles for some aspects of theatre technique.[2,3]

Wash your hands before selecting trousers and top or a dress to fit you. Washing hands, as you know, is a basic tenet of infection control but it is still the best way to remove any pathogens which you may have picked up in your passage through the hospital.

## Hats

Select the appropriate hat to completely cover your hair (men with beards are provided for as special theatre hats will cover their beards). You will be advised about the appropriate colour of hat to signal to others that you are new to theatres. (This is not a status symbol but is to indicate to surgeons, for example, that you cannot be expected to know where things are or be able to respond quickly as a team member in an emergency.)

Remove any jewellery not completely covered by your theatre clothes. Stud earrings and wedding rings are permitted though most people will remove even those when **scrubbed**. If you are not used to wearing uniform when you first come to the department you may find all this a bit trying but it is good hygiene which is the basis of good operating room technique.There is no mystique about removing either staff or patient jewellery. It can get lost or scratch people so it is better put away in a safe place.

Put your hat on before pulling your top over your hair. Hair will grow 'bugs' even if you only washed it last night. They are mostly non-pathogenic yeasts which settle out of the air but this practice helps to protect your top from possible contamination.

Hairs in a wound can cause sinus formation so this is one reason advanced for shaving patients pre-operatively. Shaving is not the best way to prevent this or to reduce post-operative infection risk.

*Activity*

Once you are settled into the department you might like to do a small literature search on the recommended methods and timing for carrying out pre-operative depilation of the patient's skin. Consider also whether these guidelines are being followed in all departments of your hospital. If not, what are the reasons?

## Shoes

Lastly, put on your theatre shoes. These will probably be washable clogs and they should have a strap around the heel to safeguard the wearer from walking out of them if he or she has to move backwards, when lifting a patient, for example. You may be given 'visitors' shoes if you are only in the theatre for a day but do make sure that they are comfortable if you are going to be in theatre for some hours. If you are to work in theatre permanently you will be given your own shoes. Most people write their name on the back of their clogs so you can use this as a guide to help you to find out and remember people's names. Overshoes should be avoided as protection is questionable and putting them on tends to contaminate your hands.[4]

This is the key time to wash your hands, after you have touched your shoes and before you go through into the theatre area. The one place which is always regarded as potentially infected is the floor and shoes go on the floor.

## Masks

It is not necessary to wear a mask until you enter a theatre where an operation is in progress or go into a room where sterile material or equipment is exposed. A minority of operating theatres have begun to give up wearing masks to protect the wound from infection as there is little researched evidence of the effectiveness of the practice.[2] However, increased awareness of the incidence of bloodborne infections has meant that the wearing of masks is regarded as staff protection as well as patient protection.[5] We shall explore this further in the 'infection control' section.

Donning and removing a mask must be done properly as, once worn, it is potentially infected and must be carefully disposed of.

### Donning a mask

1. Remove mask from box, handling by the tapes only.
2. Ensure that the mask fits snuggly across the nose. Some masks have a plastic band which can be moulded to fit.
3. Tie top tapes on the top of your head.
4. Tie the bottom tapes around your neck.
5. The mask should fit closely and comfortably.
6. Do not touch or 'wiggle' your mask.

### Removing a mask

1. Remove by the tapes only and drop straight into the rubbish bin.
2. Do not crumple your mask in your hand.
3. Do not put your used mask in your pocket.
4. Do not allow the mask under your chin.

Wearing a mask in this way will ensure that it provides effective protection for you and that you do not disseminate your own micro-organisms around the environment.

You are now ready to enter the clean environment of the operating theatre.[6]

You may find other types of masks or face protection being worn to protect individuals from noxious substances which may be inhaled in certain situations.

## Communicating in theatre

When you first work in the theatre you may experience some difficulty in hearing what people are saying behind a mask. We forget how much we understand from actually seeing people's faces. Some people feel that they are being shouted at when they come to theatres. This may be because the staff compensate, unconsciously, for wearing masks. It is, of course, possible that you will work in a theatre where masks are not worn, though this is less likely since the advent of **universal precautions** (see p 24).

*Activity*

Discuss with your clinical supervisor the reasons for not wearing masks and compare this with situations in which it is essential to wear masks, visors or eye protection.

How does the wearing of masks affect the patient's perceptions and the ability of staff to communicate with the patient?

## The theatre staff

Operating departments are staffed by nurses and other staff members who have been trained to work specifically in this area of the hospital. They all share certain skills and work together as a team with the surgeons and anaesthetists to ensure high quality patient care.

### Nurses

Most nurses who work in the operating department have completed a post registration theatre or anaesthetic course or they may have developed their specialist skills by less formal training and experience. There may be two separate teams of nurses in a large department as nurses also staff the recovery room. The recovery room nurses may have completed an anaesthetic and recovery or ITU course.

In addition to sharing the theatre skills of ODAs (see below), the nurses are responsible for planning patient care to meet the identified needs of the patient during the peri-operative period.

### Operating department assistants

Over the last 20 years or so the technicians who work solely in operating departments have been known as operating department assistants (ODAs).They complete a two year City and Guild course. Although trained in all aspects of theatre work, there has been a tendency for them to work with the anaesthetist whilst nurses have, more commonly, worked with the surgeon. They may now have been given a different name in your operating department so do find out about this.

### Operating department practitioners

The Bevan Report[7] identified some anomalies in the skill mix and roles of nurses and ODAs in theatres. Though 70% of theatre staff were nurses, only 11% of their time was spent on nursing tasks. Because of the tendency to specialise in specific areas, staffing to meet patient needs was being made more difficult as nurses and ODAs were not interchangeable within the team, despite the fact that they had completed courses covering all aspects of operating department work.[7,8] As a result one of the first NVQ schemes off the ground in health care has been the operating department practitioner scheme open to both nurses, on a 'fast track' system, and to inexperienced people by means of a two year course.[9]

All of these people will be working together in the theatre team and you may not, at first, be aware to which group a person belongs. It is unwise to assume that a man is an ODA and a woman is a nurse as an increasing number of women are looking to ODA training and there has always been a high ratio of male nurses working in operating departments. You may also see some nurses and ODAs who are working in rather specialised advanced practice roles , such as 'first assistant' to the surgeon, specific roles in transplant teams, pain control nurse, **pump technician**.[10]

There will be support for the qualified theatre staff from operating department orderlies (ODOs) who are responsible for theatre portering and patient transport and there may be some nursing auxiliaries. Both of these groups are in the process of transition to **Health Care Assistants** (HCAs), by way of Level 2 NVQ training in the same way as the ward ancillary staff.[9]

Good surgery needs good team work. In the past nurses and ODAs tended to have a separate career and management structure but this is now blending into one management structure, just as the edges of the separate training schemes and nurse education are blurring. It may be that the manager of the theatre unit you work in will be an ODA, not a nurse.

## Asking questions

You may be surprised at the amount of conversation which goes on in the theatre, or the fact that cassettes are playing. Music may be the patient's choice, if surgery is under a **local anaesthetic**, or the surgeon's during surgery under a general anaesthetic. On the other hand, the surgeon may find it difficult to concentrate if music is playing. The patient can still listen to his choice of music by using a 'Walkman' headset.

Most of the theatre team will be very happy to answer any questions you may have. Surgeons are more than ready to explain what they are doing but choose your moment carefully. It is wise to remember that patients may be able to hear and remember conversations even if they are apparently unconscious. Recent research has demonstrated long term post-operative effects from awareness during anaesthesia.[11] You should also remember that surgeon and anaesthetist carry total responsibility for the patient during this time and will not appreciate being interrupted at a crucial moment.

There are conventions about interrupting the surgeon during an operation. The first of these is to talk quietly during an operation. You may find that the surgeon may join in the conversation unless he is engaged on a difficult or complicated part of the operation. Apart from such general conversation the convention is to speak to the surgeon by approaching the scrub nurse. This is especially so if you come into the theatre with a message.

## Answering the telephone

If you are in the theatre as a visitor, avoid answering the telephone. You could get involved as the middle person in a long and complicated message. As the surgeon spends quite a lot of time at the theatre table there tend to be a number of telephone messages for both him and the anaesthetist. Anaesthetists can get to the telephone comparatively easily unless they are actually intubating a patient or coping with an emergency.

Leave responsibility for calling back with the caller whenever possible but, if you do take a message, make sure that you have it right and that you get a number to call back.

*Activity*

Find out the local procedure for dealing with telephone calls, especially the protocol for leaving messages for the surgeon. Never forget to sign a message clearly, with the date and time as well.

You may come across jargon or medical phrases you have not heard before whilst in the department. This is one of those closed environments with its own language. If you do not understand, ask! You will also find that, especially when scrubbed, theatre staff and surgeons use non-verbal cues, pointing or holding up an item, such as a suture pack, to show a colour code. People also use their eyes to indicate in which direction you will find something, rather than giving you a verbal answer if it is a time when it is important to be quiet.

## Geography of an operating theatre

You may be in a large theatre unit with many theatres and support services or you may be working in a small single or twin theatre suite. Whatever the design, all theatres have certain features in common.[6]

### Barriers

These vary from a red line on the floor to a solid wall. Barriers are not always as rigidly observed as they used to be and you may find that the only place in which it is important to wear theatre clothes, masks and shoes is in the operating theatre itself. This allows relatives, especially parents of small children, to accompany the patient as far as the anaesthetic room. You must be guided by the local rules and must obey any notices.

## Clean and dirty areas

Everything which comes into the theatre must be clean and, ideally, clean or sterile items should come directly into the clean areas, be used and then go out for disposal or recycling via 'dirty' exits and corridors. Sterile packs have outside dust covers which are removed to leave a sterile pack, double wrapped, which is then safely stored inside the clean area of the operating department.

Staff are not usually discarded but are recycled by washing and changing their clothes! Of course, you cannot sterilise or disinfect people so the one area in which the principle of **antisepsis**, as opposed to **asepsis**, still rules is skin antisepsis. This term covers both 'scrubbing up' to clean the hands of the staff and 'prepping' the patient's operation site before the incision is made.

## Operating theatre layout

Operating theatres are built on principles enshrined in government 'Building Notes'.[12] The entire unit may be built from scratch, customised, or there are standard units which can be fitted into existing buildings. The latest theatre design has modular units fitted into a large open plan building[13] with ceiling mounted fittings and swing doors. Whatever the broad design, the basic layout of an operating suite will include the same basic rooms: anaesthetic room, scrub-up, preparation room and operating theatre itself and the same basic equipment (Fig. 2.1).

## Ventilation of an operating theatre

All operating suites have a separate **ventilation system** which pumps clean, filtered air into the cleanest part of the theatre. The air pressure inside the theatre will be at a higher pressure than outside, positive pressure, so that air always flows away from the operating site and out of the theatre. This prevents contaminated air from the rest of the hospital site getting into the theatre. Most commonly used systems change the air about 25 times an hour but theatres which need to be exceptionally clean, such as orthopaedic theatres, may have special

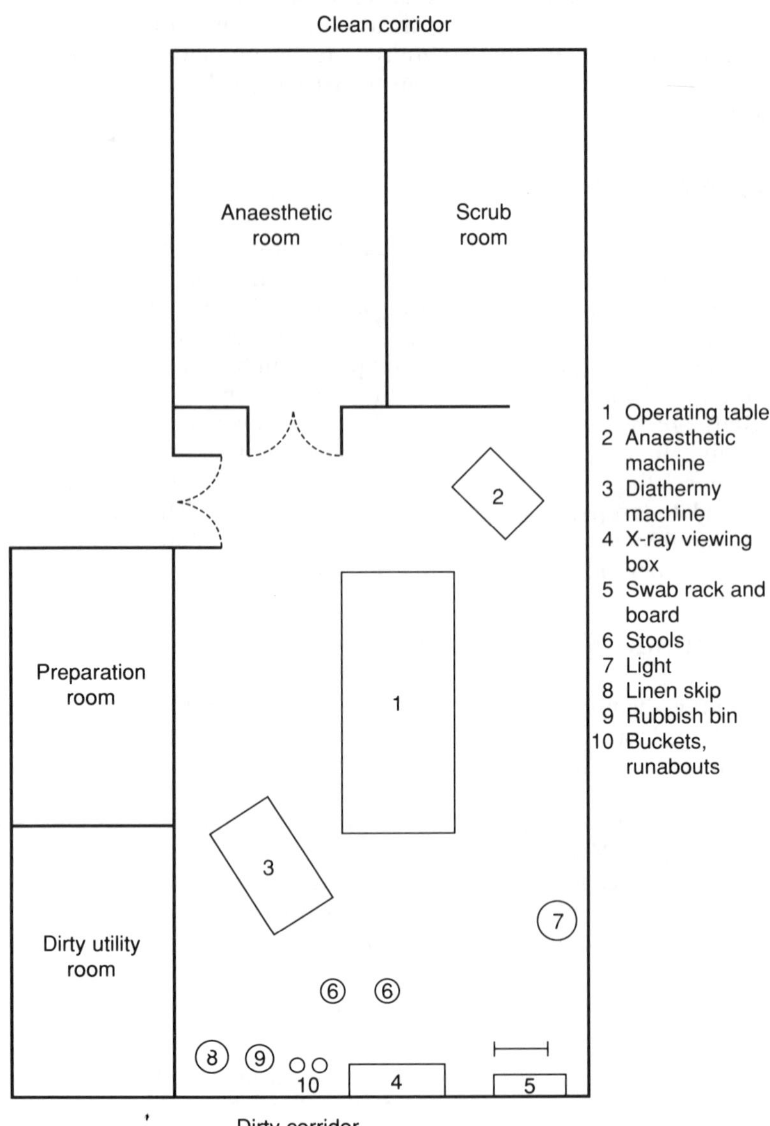


**Figure 2.1** Layout of an operating theatre. In an older theatre without CSSD back-up, there are autoclaves, sluice and more storage space.

**laminar** air systems which blow streams of air down across the patient, changing the total air in the theatre up to 300 times an hour. (Yes, it can be a trifle draughty.) Engineers and microbiologists are responsible for maintaining the efficiency of such systems by checking the **particle counts** of the air and checking and changing the filters as part of planned maintenance of the department and equipment.[6]

## Humidity and temperature

The control of air humidity is important to prevent the build-up of static and prevent the risk of sparking. Relatively high humidity levels (40–50%) also help to reduce microbial counts. We do not use many inflammable or explosive gases in modern operating theatres nowadays but we do still use volatile liquids such as spirit and alcohol as cleaning and **disinfectant** agents. Control of both humidity and temperature is important to ensure a comfortable environment for staff and patients. For the newborn or the very elderly patient we need to increase the environmental temperature. Patients for open heart surgery need a very cool environment which can be too chilly for staff comfort, especially if you are observing rather than working as part of the team.[14]

## Gas scavenging systems

The danger of the build-up of anaesthetic gases was recognised long before the introduction of **COSHH regulations**.[14] As a result the expired gases of the patients are extracted from the theatre by means of **scavenger systems**. This reduces the risk of some conditions whose incidence has been linked to exposure to anaesthetic gases.

There are one or two other preventive measures in relation to possible hazards from substances used in the operating department.

### *Activity*

If there is any danger to a baby from anaesthetic gases it will be early in a pregnancy. If you are pregnant, especially during the first trimester, you should think twice about whether you wish to be exposed to anaesthetic agents and should discuss any possible risks with your clinical supervisor or your tutor.[15] You can then decide whether you wish to work in the operating department at this time.

## Fume cabinets

Following the introduction of the COSHH regulations and awareness of the dangers of exposure to toxic substances, it has been necessary to introduce **fume cabinets** to some operating departments. The reason for this is that some advanced equipment, such as **endoscopes**, is not always heat tolerant and cannot be steam autoclaved. Though it is now a recommendation that heat sterilisation should be the method of choice, many existing instruments still have to be disinfected using substances such as **glutaraldehyde**. Do not become involved in filling or emptying containers of liquids such as glutaraldehyde until you have been educated in the proper use of protective masks and other procedures. Peak exposures during emptying and filling can be very high.[16]

## Difficult situations

Occasionally an unexpected problem crops up which can interfere with your enjoyment of working in the operating department. All of these should be discussed with your clinical supervisor or your tutor.

### Fainting

Fainting at the sight of your first operation is a theatre myth of long standing. Not true! People faint for much more mundane reasons: no breakfast (hypoglycaemia), standing still too long, getting too hot or tension from being in a new place. The same sorts of reasons which make guardsmen faint at the Trooping of the Colour!

*Activity*

1. Eat breakfast.
2. Flex your calf muscles if standing still for a long time.
3. Do tell your clinical supervisor if you have a tendency to faint.

If you feel 'funny' (you usually start to feel hot and sick) go out of theatre and sit down. A cup of tea or a glass of water may help. Of course, there will always be some wag who tells you, 'If you must faint, fall backwards. Don't contaminate the patient'.

### Claustrophobia

Quite a number of operating theatres have no windows. Working in a windowless environment with an unaccustomed cap and mask can feel very strange and confusing. Most people get used to this quickly but just a few people suffer from real claustrophobia and may need to get out of theatre until they are acclimatised. Once again, speak to your supervisor.

## References


1. NATN (1988) *Principles of Safe Practice in the Operating Theatre*. NATN, Harrogate.
2. Orr, NWN (1981) Is a mask necessary in the operating theatre? *Ann Roy Coll Surgeons England*, **63**, 390–391.
3. Moylon, N (1986) Importance of gown and drape barriers in the reduction of post-operative wound infection. *NatNews*, June, **23**(6), 10–13.
4. Humphreys, H *et al.* (1991) Theatre overshoes do not reduce operating theatre floor bacterial counts. *J Hospital Infection*, **17**, 117–123.
5. Duthie, GS *et al.* (1988) Eye protection, HIV and orthopaedic surgery. *Lancet*, **1**(8583), 481–482.
6. Brigden, R (1988) *Operating Theatre Techniques*, 5th Edn. Churchill Livingstone, Edinburgh.
7. Bevan, PG (1989) R*eport of the Working Party on the Management and Utilisation of Operating Departments*. HMSO, London.
8. Johnson, G (1991) Non-nursing duties in theatre. *BJ Theatre Nursing*, Pt. 1: **1**(3), 24–25; Pt. 2: **1**(4), 20–22.
9. Greaves, K (1993) National Vocational Qualifications rationalised. *BJ Theatre Nursing*, **3**(3) (suppl.), 13–27.
10. United Kingdom Central Council (1992) *The Scope of Professional Practice. A Position Statement*. UKCC, London.
11. Ball, K (1992) Message. *AORN J*, November, 824–827.
12. NHS Estates (1991) *Health Building Note 26. Operating Department*. HMSO, London.
13. Editorial (1992) Progress report on 'The Barn'. *B J Theatre Nursing*, **2**(5), 14–15.
14. Health and Safety Executive (1988) *Control of Substances Hazardous to Health (COSHH)*. HSE, London.
15. Vessey, MP (1978) Epidemiological studies of the occupational hazards of anaesthesia. A review. *Anaesthesia*, **33**, 430.
16. Health and Safety Executive (1993) EH40/93. *Occupational Exposure Limits, 3–4*. HSE, London.

# 3 Theatre Nursing Practice

Having managed the first hurdle of gaining access to the department, you are now ready to find out what really goes on behind the closed doors!

This chapter will focus on nursing activities within the operating room. At first you may find it difficult to associate activities within the theatre with nursing, or indeed patient care, but just remember that everything revolves around the patient, who is of prime importance, the nursing role being to ensure and maintain a safe environment during this vulnerable time of care.

Ensuring a safe environment starts with preparation. There is a vast amount of equipment within the operating theatre which needs to be checked and prepared according to the patient's individual need. Many of the preparatory duties may be delegated to other members of the theatre team, but it is a nursing responsibility to ensure everything that is needed is available and functions properly. Likewise, environmental cleanliness and control is vital to prevent avoidable complications.

*Activity*

What measures are taken to ensure environmental control? Find out what the normal parameters should be. Try to identify why these parameters might need to be adjusted for particular patients.

## Preparing the sterile field

Having checked the environment, the threatre nurse will then begin to prepare the instruments and equipment for surgery. This requires meticulous attention to detail. The aseptic techniques adopted in the theatre are, of necessity, much more rigorous than those adopted for ward dressing procedures. Trolleys are prepared in a controlled environment, by staff who have scrubbed, **gowned and gloved** according to strict protocols.[1] All equipment used within the **sterile field** must be properly sterilised and checked for efficacy before

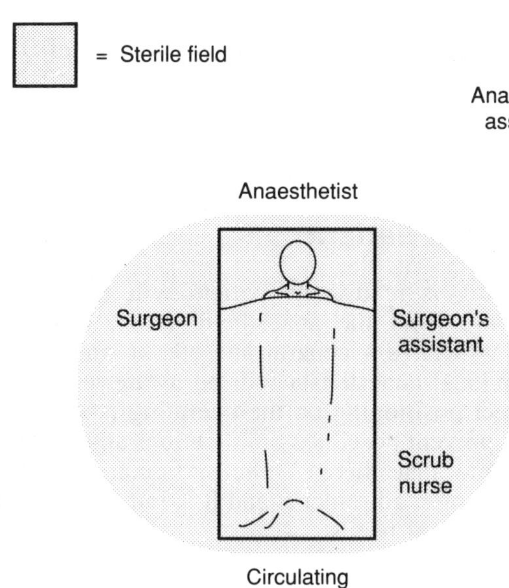


**Figure 3.1 Aseptic technique** Technique using sterile materials to prevent contamination of surgical wound by micro-organisms. Also involves antiseptic preparation of patient's skin, and hands of staff.

opening and it is the scrubbed person's responsibility to ensure the sterile field is not breached.

### *Activity*

Observe an experienced theatre nurse scrubbing, gowning and gloving. What are the protocols for this procedure?

Watch how the assistant prepares the sterile equipment and handles extra items required. How does she know that an item is sterile?

## Checks

Besides preparation of sterile equipment, the scrubbed person is responsible for controlling swabs, needles and instruments during surgery.[1,2,3] If this person is a novice, the circulating person must be a fully qualified theatre nurse, who is accountable for the patient's safety during the procedure.

*Activity*

Observe the checking procedures. At what stages of the procedure are these checks made?

How does the scrubbed person maintain control? Find out how any discrepancies are dealt with.

## Positioning the patient

When everything is ready, the patient will be transferred to the operating theatre from the anaesthetic room. Remember that not every patient will have a general anaesthetic and that those having surgery under local anaesthesia will be aware, even though usually sedated. Correct positioning on the operating table is vital to ensure patient safety, prevent possible complications and facilitate access for both surgeon and anaesthetist.[4] The particular surgery may require specific positioning requirements and it is important to anticipate and prepare for individual needs.

*Activity*

Find out when it may be necessary to place the patient in the positions listed:

Lithotomy
Supine
Prone
Lateral
Trendelenburg
Reverse Trendelenburg

Try to identify the positioning aids used for each and the particular risks/hazards of each position.[5]

When moving and handling patients, staff should also be aware of hazards to themselves and adopt safe practices to minimise back injuries.[6] There are a variety of aids that can be used in the operating theatre to facilitate this.

## Patient information

Once the patient is safely positioned, there are a number of other nursing activities which need to be initiated fairly rapidly. These will include checking the patient's identity and consent form and noting any allergies which might influence choice of skin preparation solution and wound dressings. Much of this information could be gathered in advance from a pre-operative visit by the theatre nurse.

Despite the wealth of evidence to support this practice, both in preparing the patient for the stress of surgery and gaining information which would enhance the effectiveness of care,[7,8] this is still not standard practice in many theatre suites. However, one of your objectives for this allocation might be to do some pre-operative visits or follow patients through the operating theatre; this should give you valuable insight into why particular preparations are required and why patients complain of seemingly unrelated problems post-operatively.

## Advocacy

Another important role of the theatre nurse is to be the patient's advocate, when they can no longer act for themselves or question practices. Theatre nurses have a duty to safeguard the patient's interest by speaking out about unsafe practices, ensuring that patients are treated with respect and that all information related to the patient is handled in confidence.[9] Try to put yourself or imagine someone close to you in your patient's position and treat them as you would like to be treated.

## Diathermy

During the operation the surgeon will use **diathermy** to cut or coagulate tissue, so minimising blood loss and facilitating surgery. This is a sophisticated piece of electrosurgical equipment, which is not without hazard in use.[10]

*Activity*

Find out how the diathermy works. Identify the safety measures taken to ensure the patient comes to no harm when the diathermy is in use.

Good team work is vital throughout the procedure and the scrub person needs to be vigilant, anticipating any requirements as the operation proceeds, so that surgery is not unnecessarily prolonged which would increase the risk of complications. The operating team is dependent on competent circulating assistance to provide extra sterile swabs, needles and equipment, participate in formal checking procedures, monitor blood loss, care for specimens and ensure all nursing documentation is completed.

*Activity*

Find out how specimens are handled. Try to identify the possible consequences of incorrect preservation/labelling.

What nursing documentation is completed in your theatre? Why is it important to ensure the theatre register is correctly completed?

How are used swabs counted in your theatre? How is blood loss estimated?

## Infection control

Throughout the surgery, high standards of infection control are essential, both for the patient's safety and staff protection.[11,12,13] Because of the high risk of contamination from body fluids, universal precautions must be taken when handling any contaminated items.[14,15] This means:

Treating every patient as a potential risk.
Identifying high risk surgery.
Wearing protective clothing when there is a risk of splashing or aerosol contamination.
Always wearing gloves when handling contaminated items.
Disposing of contaminated equipment according to national guidelines.
Reprocessing instruments according to national guidelines.
Ensuring sharp instruments are safely disposed of.
Mopping up all spillages, using gloves and disposable towels, as soon as they occur.
Vigilant hand washing procedures before and after any nursing activity.

Only by observing these procedures will we ensure that all patients are treated without discrimination and both staff and patient cross-infection risks are minimal.

## Hazards

Other potential risks for staff in theatre are from use of X-rays, lasers and use of substances hazardous to health.[1,6] Legislation and national guidelines are designed to protect individuals, but we also have a duty to protect ourselves.

### *Activity*

Find out what procedures there are in your theatre to ensure your safety. Do these conform to the requirements of recent legislation?

Identifying the nursing **role** in theatre and encouraging you to reflect on what you see, will, we hope, help you realise what a vital role this is and how competent practice can benefit individual patients, contributing to the success rate of surgery and ultimate patient outcomes. Because of our vigilance in providing and maintaining a safe environment, most surgery is completed without hazard. However, if an accident does occur whilst the patient is in the operating theatre, this must be reported to a senior person and fully documented.

*Activity*

Find out what procedures are followed if an accident should occur.

## References

1. NATN (1988) *Principles of Safe Practice in the Operating Theatre.* NATN, Harrogate. (Sections: E2 Lasers, E3 Diathermy, E6 Infection Control, E7 Radiation Protection, C4 Scrubbing, Gowning and Gloving, C5 The Count, C9 Universal Precautions.)
2. ACORN (1992) Counting of sponges, swabs, instruments and needles. *ACORN J*, **22**(1), 31.
3. AORN (1990) Recommended practices: sponge, sharps and instrument counts. *AORN J*, **51**(3), 838–844.
4. Anderton, JM, Keen, R and Neave, R. (1988) *Positioning The Surgical Patient.* Butterworth, London.
5. Walsh, J (1993) Post op effects of OR positioning. *RN* February, 50–58.
6. Health and Safety Executive (1988) *Control of Substances Hazardous to Health Regulations 1988 and Approved Codes of Practice.* HMSO, London.
7. Kalideen, D (1991) The case for preoperative visiting. *BJ Theatre Nursing*, Aug., vol (**5**), 19-22.
8. Caunt, H (1992) Preoperative nursing interventions to relieve stress. *BJ Nursing*, **1**(4), 171–174.
9. United Kingdom Central Council (1992) *Code of Professional Conduct.* UKCC, London.
10. Wicker, P (1992) Making sense of electrosurgery. *N Times*, **88**(45), 31–33.
11. Goodland, J (1989) Understanding hepatitis B. *N Times*, **85**(24), 69–71.
12. Kalideen, D and Edwards, S (1991) Dealing with HIV in the operating theatre. *Nursing*, **4**(42), 18–22.
13. Bowell, B (1993) Preventing infection and its spread. *Surgical Nurse*, **6**(2), 5–12.
14. Scale, T (1991) Protection of staff from body fluids. *BJ Theatre Nursing*, **1**(3), 19–21.
15. Taylor, M (1992) Universal precautions in the operating department. *Technic*, October, 6–9.

## Further reading

Booth, K (1991) Preoperative visiting: a step by step guide. *B J Theatre Nursing*: Pt. 1 Oct. 30–31; vol **1**(7) Pt. 2. Nov 6–7 vol **1**(8).

Chitwood, L and Swain, D (1992) *Perioperative Nursing: A Study and Learning Tool*. Springhouse, Pennsylvania.

Dawson, B (1988) Behind closed doors. *N Times*, **84**(41), 63–66.

Haugh, C (1993) Manual handling: a review of the new legislation. *B J Theatre Nursing*, March, vol **2**(12) 4–6.

Houghton, K (1988) Local anaesthesia. *N Times*, **84**(41), 71–75.

Hill, PD (1992) Lasers and the theatre nurse. *B J Theatre Nursing*, **1**(10), 18–19.

Ivey, D (1987) Local anaesthesia: implications for the perioperative nurse. *AORN J* **45**(3), 682–689.

Jones, H (1987) Code of conduct: human folly. *N Times*, **83**(49), 34–36.

Medical Defence Union (1988) *Theatre Safeguards*. MDU, London.

Milner, D (1987) Patient positioning: applying the nursing process. *AORN J*, **45**(5), 1117–1127.

Pediani, R (1993) Hazards and safety in theatre. *B J Theatre Nursing*, March, vol **2**(12) 19–21.

Wicker, P (1991) *Working with Electrosurgery*. NATN, Harrogate.

# 4 The Patient for Surgery

You will have probably realised by this time that many patient needs and nursing actions in the peri-operative period can be classified under:

- safety needs
- maintaining the airway
- pain control
- maintaining fluid balance
- alleviating anxiety.

You have almost certainly considered some implications of pre-operative anxiety before but perhaps not from quite this viewpoint. Early research into patient anxiety tended to relate to the relief of physical symptoms and reduction of post-operative complications. Boore[1] showed that good pre-operative preparation and explanations not only reduced anxiety levels but reduced length of stay in hospital due to the reduction in complications such as post-operative infection. Hayward's study of the relationship between good explanations and post-operative pain perceptions showed a positive correlation.[2]

*Activity*

It has been recognised for years that controlling the response to psychological stress enables the body to cope more effectively with physical stress.[3] The major reason for giving a premedication is to reduce pre-operative stress. You may wish to discuss this with colleagues. Find out why they think that premedications are given.

You will almost certainly find some people who still believe that a premedication is given to dry up secretions so that the patient will not be at risk of aspirating secretions whilst unconscious. A moment's thought will be sufficient to make you realise that atropine for this reason can be given intravenously in the anaesthetic room. The anaesthetic regimes used today are also very different.

Make a note of any unwanted side effects of the medication used. Specially notice any post-operative nausea and vomiting. Could you relate this to any specific medicine or procedure? Had the patient been particularly anxious at any time? How was the nausea or vomiting treated? Did the patient have a prophylactic antiemetic?[4]

*Activity*

Choose a patient, preferably not one for whom you are writing a theatre care study, and write up the total medication regime from premedication to post-operative pain control.

Establish why the patient was given each medicine or agent and describe the dose and effect on the patient.

This activity could be carrried out if you are allocated to work with an anaesthetist or if you have an opportunity to follow patients through their peri-operative experience.

## Pre-operative visits

Pre-operative visits are carried out in many operating departments. This is a time when patient assessment can be carried out but it has been recognised that the routine of an operating department has not always favoured the development of effective nursing practice in this area.[5] Indeed, the advance of day care surgery and the pressure on hospital beds has meant that patients are often not admitted until just before the time of their operation or they are admitted directly to a day procedure unit.

For many years, theatre nurses justified their need to visit pre-operatively by quoting anecdotal evidence of how they were able to relieve patient anxiety, how pleased the patient was to see them again in theatre reception, how the patient stated that it helped them so much.

West[6] quotes a conversation with a patient in which she describes the two nurses who had been 'special' to her as being the theatre nurse (in the anaesthetic room) and the nurse who had looked after her in the intensive care unit.

*Activity*

Discuss with your tutor the experiences you have had in reducing patient anxiety pre-operatively.

Was a pre-operative visit helpful to the patient and/or the nurse? Is someone who visits only for a few minutes the right person to help a patient cope with their anxiety?

On the other hand, is the nurse who was with the patient, giving the patient undivided attention, at a time of great stress going to be the one remembered as someone 'special'?

Anxiety is the product of helplessness.[7] Recent research has concentrated on empowering the patient as a way of helping patients to cope with the ordeal of surgery. This calls for nurses to reduce the amount of control they exercise over their patients and to help the patients to see that they can control some of the things which are happening to them. One suggested means of empowering the patient is to 'teach' him or her.[8] Unfortunately, in inexpert or thoughtless hands this can become 'telling' rather than sharing.[9] Establishing a therapeutic relationship means recognising a patient's rights, strengths and self-knowledge rather than their weaknesses and needs.[10]

The therapeutic relationship is about sharing knowledge and information, rather than telling and is also about an **empathic** understanding of the patient's feelings, beliefs and coping mechanisms.

Despite public lip service paid to patients' rights and choices the present high cost of health care, at a time of economic stringency, has resulted in a rapid passage through the surgical experience for most patients. Avis carried out a study of a group of patients having day surgery in Nottingham.[11] He concluded that the system did not allow for much choice or patient participation though there was a high degree of patient satisfaction. He also concludes that patients do not expect autonomy and participation in their relationships with health professionals. He identifies three main attitudes amongst the people he interviewed which can be described as:

1. 'Being told' – not up to me to ask or initiate questions. The patients expected to be passive.
2. 'Going to get it fixed' – rather like taking the car to the garage. This depersonalisation abdicates responsibility to the carers.
3. 'Letting them get on with it'– patients expect to be told what to do.

Some recent research by Meredith[12] would indicate that patient participation and autonomy will only improve if the implicit message is changed. More effective communication could be achieved by sharing the information and consenting procedures.

### *Activity*

In view of what we believe about patient autonomy and how important it is to share information with patients, discuss whether you think these attitudes are part of the patient's coping mechanisms.

Avis suggests that being a 'work object' may act as a defence against the indignities, intrusions and frightening nature of modern medical treatment. In fact, we probably get used to most patients adopting these sorts of attitudes to distance themselves from what is happening to them on admission to hospital, when they are very ill or when they are about to go to theatre.

*Activity*

What tends to happen if carers are confronted by a patient who asks questions and has a strong need to know and control what is happening to him or her? Sometimes, such a patient is labelled as 'difficult'. Next time you see something like this happening you could carry out a critical incident analysis. Try also to establish an open relationship without resenting the patient's need to know. It may be part of the patient's personality but there may be deeper anxieties than those concerned only with the operation.

In the final analysis all patients admitted for surgery arrive in the **anaesthetic room**. Most of them are awake, though some may be more or less sleepy. They are surrounded by a team of competent health care professionals. You, as the nurse, must respond to a patient's need for support rapidly. This is a time when you have to establish an immediate rapport and when you need to go more than half way to meet the other person, your patient. Basic human communication skills are what is needed.

Look at the patient. Smile and use their name and when it comes to the point of the injection, hold the patient's hand. You will know you have done the right thing by the pressure of the response. You will have humanised a frightening experience.

## References

1. Boore, JPR (1978) *Prescription for Recovery*. RCN, London.
2. Hayward, J (1975) *Information – A Prescription against Pain*. RCN, London.
3. Boore, JPR (1976) An investigation into the effect of some aspects of pre-operative preparation of patients on post-operative stress and recovery. Unpublished PhD thesis, University of Manchester.
4. Thompson, J (1992) Post-operative nausea and vomiting. *BJ Theatre Nursing*, **2**(7), 22–24.
5. Astbury, C (1988) *Stress in Theatre Nursing*. Scutari Press, London.
6. West, BJM (1993) Caring, the essence of theatre nursing. *BJ Theatre Nursing*, **3**(9) (suppl), 15–26.
7. Burridge, L (1993) Challenging the traditional view of pre-operative visiting. *B J Theatre Nursing*, **3**(4), 12–15.
8. Brown, A (1992) Pre-operative teaching – a literature review. *BJ Theatre Nursing*, **2**(3) S15–S16.
9. Lindeman, CA and Van Aernam, B (1971) Nursing intervention with presurgical patients. *Nursing Res*, **20**, 319–332.
10. Devine, A (1993) Empowering the patient to control post operative pain. *B J Theatre Nursing*, **3**(3), 11–12.
11. Avis, M (1992) Silent partners. *BJ Theatre Nursing*, **2**(7), 8–11.
12. Meredith, P (1993) Patient participation in decision making and consent to treatment. The case of general surgery. *Sociology of Health and Illness*, **15**(3), 315–336.

# 5 Utilising Assessment Skills

This chapter examines the knowledge, skills and attitudes required by the theatre nurse in order to undertake assessment of the patient's needs during the peri-operative period. It also examines the issues concerned with utilising a problem solving approach.[1,2] During the activities described in the text you will be asked to examine your existing skills and to build on those in a manner that is relevant to assessing the patient in the peri-operative period.

Within this period of time there are discrete stages, which can be related to varying priorities of care needs. These can be viewed as:

**Pre-operative care** – transfer to the theatre suite from the ward; in the anaesthetic room/area.
**Intra-operative care** – on the operating table during surgery.
**Post-operative care** – transfer to, and care in, the recovery room; transfer back to the ward from the theatre suite.

The 'transfer' time may sound fairly trivial but this is where the patient passes from the care of one group of nurses to another. It is here that **communications** failures can occur.

The following activities should be discussed with your clinical supervisor whose help you will need to complete them. It may not be possible to complete all of these activities during one short placement so you may wish to be selective about which activities you complete. Decide whether you want to concentrate on activities which help you to plan patient care or whether you want to increase your understanding of how each member of the theatre team contributes to patient care. If you are allocated to the theatre or recovery room for a longer time you should be able to complete all of the activities.

## Data collection

In order to minimise the vulnerability of each and every individual passing through the operating department the assessment must involve the collection of data.[1,2] Data collection can be divided into four closely interrelated categories. They are:

1. Historical data – past history;
2. Current data – present condition;
3. Objective (quantifiable) data – nurse observed;
4. Subjective (qualitative) data – patient reported.

*Activity*

Think back to situations where you have utilised these categories of data before. How useful was it? How easy was it to obtain? Was it relevant to the current situation? What did you do with the data when you had collected it?

## Nursing accountability

Within the operating department there exists a complex multidisciplinary team with many skills. Many are experts in their own field but not all are involved in every stage of peri-operative care.

*Activity*

Make a list of all the theatre personnel, inside and outside the operating department, who contribute to the assessment process. Can you identify the unique role of the operating department nurses in identifying patient needs?

Bergman suggests that there are a number of prerequisites to practitioners being held **accountable** for prescribing care.[3] Firstly the practitioner must acquire the necessary knowledge, skills and attitudes to meet the needs of the patients. Without this knowledge the practitioner should not be accepting responsibility for prescribing the care of an individual patient.[4]

*Activity*

Talk to a number of theatre personnel of various grades and professions and identify how they have expanded their competences to a level of expertise which meets the needs of clients.[5] Have they acquired these additional qualities in an informal or formal way?

**Autonomy** is a prerequisite for a practitioner to be accountable within their scope of practice.[3] This means that nurses have an independent role symbiotic or interdependent with other members of the theatre team. Many nurses will have extended their assessment skills in order to identify the needs of the patients whom they serve. The nurse will also make the decision as to who will actually deliver the care needed to meet those needs.[5]

## Collecting data

Assessment of the patient does not take place in a vacuum. Assessment should be considered within the context of clients' needs and the environment in which the care is to be delivered as this will influence the assessment process. The physical and psychological status of an individual may influence their perceived needs. You may find it useful to refer back to Chapter 4 before you consider carrying out a pre-operative visit. You should also take time to reflect on how pre-operative visiting is achieved in your theatres.

*Activity*

When you and your clinical supervisor feel that you are ready, choose two patients, about to undergo the same operation, whose pre-operative assessment you wish to observe or assist in. Whether you will observe or assist or carry out the patient interview is going to depend on your previous experience of patient assessment both in theatres and elsewhere.

Consider the following as possible tools for assessment.

| | |
|---|---|
| A model of nursing | Sphygmomanometer and stethoscope |
| Open ended questions | Thermometer |
| Closed questions | Watch |
| Touch | Weighing scales |
| Smell | Height measurement |
| Observations | Pressure sore risk scale |
| Listening | Pain assessment scale |
| Prescription sheet | Fluid balance charts |
| | Multistix for urinalysis |

## Analysing data

Following both interviews, reflect on your findings. Include the responses made by the patient or significant others. Discuss this with your clinical supervisor and then assist in the planning of the care. How do each patient's needs differ?

*Activity*

Reflect back on the two patients that you interviewed. In what way would you suggest the patients' background, history and values influenced their perceived needs? How did you allow for this in the care plan in order to ensure delivery of care to meet the patient's individual needs?

Which of the assessment tools highlighted priority needs? Were any needs not articulated but recognised in other ways?

Consider whether you have correctly identified priority needs in view of the fact that the patient may not yet have any **nursing problems** – these may not occur until after the anaesthetic or after the operation. Will the need for reassurance then become less important?

Patients do not come to surgery without some knowledge. Past experiences influence the present situation. This can be helpful if it is accurate and informed knowledge but this is not always the case.

*Activity*

Arrange to observe an interview with a patient and attempt to identify how and why that individual is about to undergo surgery. How long had the process taken from first perceiving a problem to undergoing the present intervention? Why was this? Does this patient appear to have any preconceived ideas with regard to the possible outcomes?

Make a note of the types of misinformation that the patient may have acquired. Why do you think this has happened?

Did you feel, during the interview, that the patient was ready to take a passive role and put all his trust in those caring for him?

If it is possible, you might like to follow this up by a post-operative interview.

## Patient interviews

The environment can profoundly affect the interview/assessment process, particularly in relation to the collection of personal information. It is not in the scope of this chapter to consider the effects of the nurse's own interpersonal skills but discuss these with your clinical supervisor.

In addition to this the availability of resources can also affect the comprehensiveness of the assessment.[6,7,8]

*Activity*

Reflect back on the interviews that you have been involved in to date. How did the environment help or hinder the interview process? Did it enable you to empathise with the patient and demonstrate trust?

How did you acquire the patient data? Was it comprehensive or did you have to cut it short due to lack of time, resources or the availability of the patient?

Where you identified a deficit, decide how you could rectify this in future.

You may have found that theatre nurses are having difficulty in finding time to visit all patients pre-operatively. Can you identify ways in which they are striving to carry out this important first stage of the peri-operative nursing process?

*Activity*

Individuals who have visual and hearing deficits may rely heavily upon one mode of communication. Do you have any thoughts on how assessors communicated with such patients? Did the assessor acquire the necessary data in order to plan their care throughout the peri-operative time and was this recorded so that everyone caring for the patient was aware?

What problems may occur in the immediate post-operative period?[9]

Assessment is the first stage of the nursing process and is continuous with the other stages. No one method of data collection is comprehensive enough in isolation.

*Activity*

Reflect on all the interviews you have conducted with your clinical supervisor and make notes as to how you acquired the following:

- Past history
- Health status of client
- Knowledge, skills and beliefs
- Self-awareness

How did the use of that information influence and develop your ability to:

- Listen
- Question
- Clarify
- Measure
- Observe
- Use touch
- Interpret information
- Document your findings?

You should now have a better understanding of the importance of assessment and the complex nature of the skills required in order to undertake a comprehensive and meaningful assessment of patients undergoing surgical intervention.

## References

1. Barnett, DC and Knight, G (1987) *Patients' Problems and Plans – Nursing Care of Patients with Medical Disorders.* Edward Arnold, London.
2. McFarlane, J and Castledine, G (1982) *A Guide to the Practice of Nursing – Using the Nursing Process.* C.V. Mosby, St Louis.
3. Bergman, R (1981) Accountability – definition and dimensions. *Int Nursing Rev*, 28 February, **28**(2), 53–59.
4. United Kingdom Central Council (1992) *Code of Professional Conduct.* UKCC, London.
5. United Kingdom Central Council (1992) *Scope of Professional Practice.* UKCC, London.
6. Sawyer, J (1988) On behalf of the patient. *N Times*, **84**(41), 28–30.
7. Porter, S (1988) Siding with the system. *N Times*, **84**(41), 30–31.
8. Burnard, P (1987) Meaningful dialogue . . . elements that comprise a therapeutic conversation. *N Times*, **83**(20), 43–45.
9. Faulkner, A (1992) *Effective Interaction with Patients.* Churchill Livingstone, Edinburgh.

# 6 Preparing the Plan of Care

A plan is 'a large scale detailed map of a small area', 'a scheme for accomplishing a purpose' or 'a scheme drawn up beforehand'.[1] Planning nursing care can be viewed as all of these.

The UKCC advises nurses that 'the important activity of making and keeping records is an essential and integral part of care'. The purpose of records is to 'provide accurate, current, comprehensive and concise information concerning the condition and care of the client and associated observations'. Keeping records is also about providing a 'record of problems that arise and the action taken' and 'providing evidence of care' to justify nursing interventions.[2]

Nursing records should incorporate 'any factors that appear to affect the client', physical, psychological or social. Entries to records should be in chronological order with a rationale given to support the professional decision making process. Records will then 'support standard setting, quality assessment and **audit**' in the clinical setting. They will also be the '**baseline record** against which improvement or deterioration may be judged'.[2]

Who else can do this effectively for the patient during the peri-operative period other than a nurse based in the operating department? If patient records do not include a peri-operative care plan or, at the very least, a record of peri-operative care, they are incomplete.

### *Activity*

Identify how the records of patients you have met so far are maintained. Where are they kept before, during and following interventions? Who completes the documents, where and when?

As far as you can tell, are they accurate, current, comprehensive and concise in relation to providing the care of the specific patients?

Do the records appear to consider the physical, psychological and social needs of the client?

Are all the entries in chronological order?

Is the decision making process supported in the records?

Reflect on how the planning of care is carried out and discuss your conclusions with your supervisor. There may be some use of 'tick boxes' or check lists. Is this appropriate? Can patient care be planned from this type of information?

## Patient consent

Consent means 'a voluntary, uncoerced decision, made by a sufficiently competent, autonomous person on the basis of adequate information and deliberation, to accept rather than reject some proposed course of action'.[3] If informed consent is to be achieved it must be a mutually agreed activity and care planning must include some direction on how consent will be achieved.

*Activity*

What is meant by the terms:

- implied consent?
- verbal consent?
- written consent?

What is the nurse's role in gaining the consent of patients about to undergo surgical intervention?

A useful document for you to read to support your ideas and thoughts on this is the UKCC's *Exercising Accountability* (Section D 'Consent and Truth').[4]

You may have found that obtaining patient consent is very closely prescribed by local policy and national guidelines and is implicit rather than explicitly stated in the care plan.

## Planning patient care

The patient may have a number of identified needs or problems and, as a result, may therefore need all the skills of the multidisciplinary team. Planning enables the multidisciplinary team to identify what can be done to assist the patient. If, for example, informed consent is a goal which is to be realistically achieved, goal setting must be a mutually agreed activity. Goal setting should be aimed at identifying methods which resolve actual and potential problems.

## Written patient goals

Goal statements should identify:

- a 'performer', nurse, patient or relative, for instance, who will implement the action;

- the action to be performed;
- a change in patient behaviour which is to be accomplished or measured.

Goal statements thus allow for evaluation of achievement. Measurements obtained during the assessment phase act as a baseline for subsequent measurements.

Other factors may need to be considered in the planning phase. The following is a list of possible considerations, which may influence goal achievement and how the achievement might be measured:

- Route of admission to hospital;
- Availability of bed;
- Availability of theatre time;
- Medical diagnosis;
- Need for extra equipment, e.g. splint;
- Availability of results of diagnostic tests;
- Baseline vital signs (obtained on initial assessment);
- Physical and psychological status;
- Valid patient consent;
- Potential or perceived threats.

Goals should be realistically achievable, mutually acceptable and supportive of the patient's needs. The plan should provide consistency of care and continuity and be comprehensive. This may entail the acquisition of additional resources.

## Managing resources

Human resources, in this case the members of the theatre teams, are a major component in achieving effective, efficient and economical care. It needs careful planning to ensure their availability at the right time.

*Activity*

With your clinical supervisor identify material and human resources available to meet the needs of a patient.

Are they available in the operating department or do they need to be arranged with another department?

Will they arrive with the patient and, if so, how is this actioned and by whom will it be actioned?

## Right patient . . . right operation

One aim of the theatre nurse is to ensure that the correct patient arrives at the designated operating theatre at the correct time with correct documentation in order to ensure that they receive the correct operative procedure.[5]

*Activity*

With your clinical surpervisor check how this is consistently achieved.

Do you know where to find the theatre operating list? Where is the theatre register kept? Is there a standard check list for 'checking in' each patient arriving at the reception area?

Whose responsibility is it to complete each piece of the documentation? What is the protocol to be applied if this is not followed correctly?

Is there a procedure for sending for patients? Who is responsible for this?

Reflect on whether you now feel better prepared to become actively involved in patient care in the operating department.

## Standardised care

We should not finish this chapter without mentioning standardised or 'core' care plans. All patients have many needs in common during surgery. These 'normative' needs can be met by actions which do not need to be written out in full for every patient. Your theatre may have developed a core care plan or nursing standard statements which define how such needs are met. The individual patient care plans will, then, identify only specific needs and actions to meet those individual needs over and above the standard care.

## References

1. *Chambers English Dictionary* (1988) Cambridge University Press, Cambridge.
2. United Kingdom Central Council (1993) *Standards for Records and Record Keeping*. UKCC, London.
3. Gillon, R (1986) *Philosophical Medical Ethics*. John Wiley & Sons, Chichester.
4. United Kingdom Central Council (1989) *Exercising Accountability*. UKCC, London.
5. Medical Defence Union RCN/NATN (1986) *Theatre Safeguards*. MDU, London.

# 7 Delivering the Care

Care given according to a well written care plan has stated goals of care and defined patient outcomes by which we evaluate its effectiveness. Implementation of a nursing care plan aims to achieve stated goals. As the nurse is accountable to her patient for the quality of the care delivered, the nurse must not merely implement planned care but must continually reassess the patient and modify the plan. This is particularly so during the peri-operative period when the patient's responses to the treatment and medication may occur very quickly.

As a student you must ensure that you are capable of undertaking tasks which you are asked to perform[1] or which you may consider performing on your own initiative. Remember even registered nurses must 'acknowledge any limitations in their knowledge and competence and decline any duties or responsibilities unless able to perform them in a safe and skilled manner'.[2]

*Activity*

With your clinical supervisor select one of the care plans which you have been active in formulating and examine each of the nursing actions and the anticipated outcomes. Do you have the necessary knowledge and the appropriate skills to perform the nursing actions required in the care plan?[3]

1. Make a list of the skills which you do have.
2. What is the theory which underpins these activities?
3. Make a list of the skills you do not have.
4. Arrange with your clinical supervisor to address those deficits which are realistically and appropriately achievable by you.
5. How do you intend to prepare for these activities?

Do you need to read a text book?
Do you need to refer to the relevant standards of care?
Do you need to develop new skills before you approach a patient?
Would you prefer to see it performed by an experienced member of the team?
Do you need to involve your tutor?

As a nurse you will usually find that patients trust and respect you regardless of your status in the hierarchy. You should not abuse the privileged access to their person and property or do anything which will make a patient feel that you cannot be trusted and respected.

*Activity*

Usually the ward nurse will have dealt with the personal items, but you may receive a patient in theatre with false teeth, due to either the patient or anaesthetist requesting to keep them in. Or the patient may need their hearing aid in order to effectively communicate with members of the theatre team. With your mentor, identify the procedure to be followed to ensure the safe keeping and identification of such personal items. Consider, also, how the embarrassment or communication difficulties can be kept to a minimum. How do the theatre team deal with personal items made of metal left in situ for either spiritual or sentimental reasons (e.g. wedding rings)?

## Factors which will influence the delivery of care

The **medical diagnosis** is usually closely related to the nursing care. Within the peri-operative period this can be extremely significant. For example, a patient with a disorder of the gastrointestinal tract may not be able to tolerate an oral intake for some time, despite complaining of hunger or thirst. Such issues have been identified as essential needs to maintain life.[4,5,6]

## Resources available

### Nursing personnel

The skill mix of the department needs proactive planning, in order to meet the anticipated workload for that period. This will be influenced by the way in which nursing work is organised – team nursing, primary nursing or task allocation.[7]

Effectiveness and availability of the nursing resource can be influenced by:

- previous patient goals not achieved – emergency return to theatre;
- time taken for teaching activities – new staff member;
- sickness, holidays, absence – someone rang in sick;
- additional unidentified workload – urgent management request;
- need to deploy workforce elsewhere based on greater priority of need – urgent emergency admission(s).

*Activity*

Talk to the **team leader** or **departmental manager** and ask if any of the above could affect the care plans that you have helped to develop. Establish with this person what contingency plans there are for any of these events.

## Equipment

Equipment for an operation may be part of the furniture and fittings of a specialist theatre, e.g. orthopaedic theatres have special tables and built-in laminar air flow ventilation systems. The timing of operations may rely on a particular operating theatre being available.

Within the patient's plan of care other material items of equipment will be identified for effective and efficient delivery of care, e.g. PCA pump or an expensive piece of equipment shared by a number of surgeons.

Other factors influencing the timing of an operation are:

- demand may exceed supply;
- lack of experienced team members;
- patient withdraws consent;
- medical prescription has changed;
- change in patient status.

*Activity*

Find out the procedure for booking someone into a specialist theatre. Identify the necessary specialist equipment needed and any contingency plans for shortage of equipment, both long term and short term. Have you observed any situation in which shortage of resources affected the delivery of care to a patient?

## Environment

The operating theatre is an environment of which patients have very limited knowledge. This is because it is a place which is not open to the public. Any individual who has previously visited the operating theatre may have a very limited memory of their visit due to the medication they received as part of the anaesthetic. Surgical and anaesthetic techniques are changing. Surgery is less invasive, less debilitating and often does not require the administration of a general anaesthetic. As a result, more patients are likely to be conscious whilst in the operating theatre or wake up more rapidly following their operation.[8,9]

*Activity*

Examine the operating lists for the day or week and identify an individual patient who will not be receiving a general anaesthetic. Negotiate to be involved in their operative procedure and in so doing ask the sister/team leader/primary nurse how the theatre needs to be arranged in order to receive this patient and list the rationale behind this activity. If possible repeat this exercise for patients who have:

- a known infective condition:
- an immunosuppressive condition;
- an increased risk of hypothermia during anaesthesia.

Reflect on the ways of meeting the differing needs.

## Care delivery as a dynamic concept

This requires the practitioner to be able to:

- be alert to the many and varied characteristics of the setting;
- be aware of the range of possibilities for action;
- draw upon previous relevant experience;
- have in mind previously formulated personal theory;
- draw upon relevant theory;
- take into account the influence of personal values;
- be aware of how these personal values relate to professional frames of reference;
- make a professional judgement;
- act upon a decision;
- continually evaluate the decision and its effects.

These various facets of care delivery require the practitioner to perform 'reflection in action'. This ensures that learning is continuous and each practitioner continues to develop his or her practice.

## References

1. United Kingdom Central Council (1992) *Student's Charter*. UKCC, London.
2. United Kingdom Central Council (1992) *Code of Professonal Conduct*, 3rd edn. UKCC; London.
3. United Kingdom Central Council (1992) *Scope of Professional Practice*. UKCC, London.
4. Maslow, AH (1970) *Motivation and Personality*, 2nd edn. Harper & Row, New York.
5. Kalish, R (1983) *The Psychology of Human Behaviour*, 5th edn. Wadsworth Inc., Belmont, California.

6. Tortora, GJ (1981) *Principles of Anatomy and Physiology*, 3rd edn. Harper & Row, New York.
7. Pearson, A (1991) *Primary Nursing*. Chapman & Hall, London.
8. Rothrock, JC (1990) *Alexander's Care of the Patient in Surgery*. C.V. Mosby, St Louis.
9. Atkinson, RS, Rushman, GB and Davies, NH (1993) *Lee's Synopsis of Anaesthesia*, 11th edn. Butterworth Heinemann, London.

# 8 Evaluating the Plan of Care

Evaluation completes the cycle of nursing care. Assessment is about data collection in order that care may be prescribed. Evaluation, on the other hand, is about critically and constructively analysing the goals of the prescribed care to identify whether the **criteria** (patient outcomes) have been met from a professional point of view and, most importantly, from the patient's perspective.

According to Wilensky, accountability is paramount if practitioners are to remain autonomous. One of the criteria for a body of people calling themselves professionals is the notion of self-governance. Hence the need for the professional to evaluate the effectiveness of their actions.[1] At the same time, a partnership with the patient should be established to set mutually agreeable goals which are meaningful to both nurse and patient. Like assessment, evaluation depends upon the individual's perception of what constitutes success and quality. If consumer satisfaction is to be achieved then the patient's criteria for success, as well as those of the professional, must be met.

An additional perspective of evaluation is that of organisational accountability,[2] in relation to economy, efficiency and effectiveness of treatment, particularly in a climate where market forces are affected by financial constraints.[3] Only by undertaking regular audits will managers be able to understand the who, why, where and how of patient care delivery, in an attempt to match resources and skills to need.

For the organisation, for professionals and for individuals, evaluation may prove to be essential in identifying the reasons for deficits and surpluses in resource allocation. Resources include equipment, staff, skill mix, time and finance. Clearly and concisely documenting the intended patient outcomes will help the practitioner to justify the means.

The difficulty with evaluation is that it is subjective, depending upon the perspective of the individual undertaking the review. It is also influenced by factors intrinsic to the patient and by other extrinsic factors. The practitioner may strive to control these factors. However, when the factors influencing care are altered, so are the criteria by which care may be measured. The extrinsic factors such as environment, resources and individuals may be more readily amenable to control or influence than the intrinsic factors directly related to the patient's **homoeostatic** mechanisms.

Hunt *et al.* suggest that, for an item to be measurable, it must be stated either as:

- a behavioural response;
- a verbal response;
- a specific observation or assessment;
- a physiological measurement.[4]

These factors embrace theoretical concepts which underpin nursing practice and the practice of other health care professions. There are some factors which can be measured which we have already mentioned and which can contribute to a more objective evaluation.

### *Activity*

Refer back to the care plans with which you have been actively involved and identify which of the objective evaluation processes you may utilise to evaluate the care given. They may be any of the following:

- behavioural responses from the patient, e.g. patient demonstrates gag/swallowing reflex (to show they can guard their own airway);
- verbal responses of the patient, e.g. patient complains of pain;
- specific observation made by the nurse, e.g. respiratory rate, colour;
- physiological measurement, e.g. pulse rate, oxygen saturation.

This will require the practitioner to compare the goals stated with the actual outcomes. Any discrepancies should then be documented in the patient's notes.

You may notice, at this point, that working in a multidisciplinary team may lead to conflicts about where patient information is to be charted.

### *Activity*

Reflect on how this has been solved so that different groups of professionals may share the same records and yet complete specific records which are relevant to their own area of accountability. You may find it particularly interesting to consider how the anaesthetists and recovery nurses have addressed this problem.[5]

Evaluation requires nurses and patients to stand in judgement of the care given and should always be written down. This will enable continuity of care (the ward nurses will have a theatre record) and consistency of care (theatre nurses can refer to such records in implementing future care plans).[5]

The recordings should be specific and include date, time, place and by whom and how the evaluation was conducted. This then leads the practitioner into the next cycle of care – reassessment of needs and resetting goals in the light of the current findings.

There is a problem here for peri-operative nurses. Patients are not always in a fit state to be involved in reassessment. However, retrospective evaluation can be carried out with conscious patients or at post-operative visits.

*Activity*

In making the comparisons between the intended and the actual outcomes identify any of the goals that were not measurable. If any of the objectives were not measurable which ones were they:

- physiological outcomes?
- psychological outcomes?
- sociological outcomes?
- spiritual outcomes?

Reflect on your finding for a moment and list the reasons why you think there are discrepancies between the intended and actual outcomes. Discuss your notes and see if your supervisor agrees with you. If not, do you think their explanation was valid?

*Activity*

Where the outcomes did not match the goals, what happened?

- Was there renegotiation of care with the client?
- Had the goals been unrealistic?
- Was there a lack of resources?
- Was there a sudden and unexpected change in the patient's status?

Reflect on how reassessment was carried out during the patient's stay in the operating department and discuss with your supervisor how and why this differs from reassessment in other situations.

## Modifying care plans

You have now reviewed all the stages of care planning in the operating department context and seen how care planning is modified in a very different setting. Evaluating the effectiveness of care during one patient episode may not have any effect on the care of that particular patient. A key issue will be recording the care given as the care of the patient will now pass to another group of nurses.

The UKCC states that care plans are only of use if they are up to date.[5] Patient status changes rapidly in critical care areas and actions by the team happen so quickly that reassessment and evaluation are constant but not recorded in great detail. Planning is something you do for events in the future, not for something you are doing now.

### *Activity*

Reflect on how the use of standardised care plans assists in planning ahead for the care of patients during the peri-operative period.

Has this resulted in the development of protocols and procedures so that the pre-, intra- and post-operative care of patients is carried out smoothly and efficiently?

Read through the records which accompany the patient from the department and decide whether this is a true record of the treatment and care given.

The next chapter considers two care studies of patients. The first thing to remember is that these care plans were developed by nurses as educational exercises. In doing these studies a nurse steps back to look at their work and practice from a different perspective. It is a way to learn both about the patient experience and about care planning.

Those students who have insufficient time to carry out care planning during their placement in the operating department may wish to complete some of the activities in this chapter on the following care plans.

## References


1. Wilensky, HL (1964) Professionalisation of everyone. *Am J Sociol,* **70**, 137–158.
2. Rhodes, B (1983) Accountability in nursing – alternative perspectives: part 1. *N Times*, **13**, 65–66.
3. NHS (1983) *National Health Management Inquiry*. HMSO, London.
4. Marks Maran, DJ and Hunt, J (1986) *Nursing Care Plans – The Nursing Process*, 2nd edn. John Wiley & Sons, Chichester.
5. United Kingdom Central Council (1993) *Standards for Records and Record Keeping*. UKCC, London.

# 9 The Peri-operative Process

In this chapter, we will show you how nurses use the skills of assessment, planning, implementation and evaluation when caring for real patients during the peri-operative period.

All the information in this section was gathered by practising theatre nurses during the course of their daily work and is the result of assessing the individual needs of genuine patients requiring surgical intervention (confidentiality has been maintained by the use of a pseudonym and omitting any details which could identify the patient or hospital).

The examples chosen illustrate how the use of different theoretical models can influence how we gather and utilise information gained during a pre-operative assessment and how different philosophical perspectives will govern the way we organise nursing activities to meet individual patient care needs. These are not complete care plans. The first plan is pre-operative, the second post-operative care.

*Activity*

To fully appreciate how nurses have used theoretical models to plan care, you will need to read up on these.

The reading list at the end of the chapter should provide enough background information so that you can follow the assessment and planning stages.

## Using Roper *et al.*'s model[1] to plan care for Mrs Oakley who is to undergo surgery for breast reconstruction

Mrs Oakley, a 55 year old married lady, was admitted to hospital for a breast reconstruction following a segmented resection of her left breast for carcinoma two years previously. Prior to her surgery, she had worked full time as a badminton coach, but had found it increasingly difficult to continue due to restricted arm movement. She was also disappointed with her scar, which she described as 'puckered' and 'looked ugly'. Mrs Oakley had not realised that there were specially made silastic prostheses for use following a segmented resection and had been without for the first 18 months following her surgery. When she had discovered that there were such prostheses, she had been a lot happier about her clothing.

Mrs Oakley had a positive outlook, with good family support. She was determined to put her illness behind her and get back to work.

Using the activities of living, an initial assessment was made from which a plan of care was devised.

By assessing and planning to meet real and potential problems, the theatre nurse can ensure that each patient receives safe care without neglecting their individual needs.

The following shows how Mrs Oakley's care was implemented during the intraoperative phase.

Mrs Oakley was collected for theatre by the theatre nurse who had undertaken her pre-operative assessment. This ensured continuity of care, provided Mrs Oakley with psychological support and allowed the nurse to monitor all preventative and protective measures taken to maintain her safety. The nurse was able to provide support during the induction of anaesthesia, reiterating and reinforcing pre-operative education.

Once anaesthetised, Mrs Oakley was transferred to the theatre and carefully placed onto the operating table. She was placed in the supine position with her left arm extended on an arm board so that the surgeon could have good access to the left breast and axilla. Both arms were padded with gamgee before securing to prevent pressure which could cause nerve damage. Mrs Oakley was on a heated ripple mattress to prevent pressure sores and loss of body heat during a lengthy surgical procedure. Her body temperature was also monitored throughout the procedure by means of a rectal temperature probe. The diathermy plate was secured to the right thigh in the correct manner to ensure the circuit was complete and electrosurgery could be used safely.

Mrs Oakley was catheterised with a size 16 FG Foley catheter attached to a urimeter to ensure an empty bladder during the procedure and to enable accurate output recording, necessary for the anaesthetist to maintain an adequate fluid replacement.

Because of Mrs Oakley's high risk of deep vein thrombosis, Flowtron boots were applied to her lower limbs during the operation, over the antiembolism stockings which remained in situ until Mrs Oakley was able to mobilise.

Throughout the surgery the circulating nurse works with other members of the team to provide a safe environment. This involves attending to the needs of the surgical team in providing extra sterile equipment as necessary and being vigilant for any changes occurring throughout the procedure, adjusting the settings on the electrosurgical

**ASSESSMENT OF ACTIVITIES OF LIVING**

**DATE** – 7.6.93

| AL | USUAL ROUTINES<br>What he/she can or cannot do independently | PATIENTS PROBLEMS<br>Actual/Potential<br>P = Potential |
|---|---|---|
| 1. **Breathing** | Gave up smoking many years ago. Scarring on chest wall and past therapy has caused pain on deep inspiration. | P = Chest Infection |
| 2. **Eliminating** | No problems with micturition. Bowels open daily and no problems since the ?ulcerative colitis/?irritable bowel syndrome over 20 years ago. | |
| 3. **Maintaining a Safe Environment** | No problems with self-care even with chest scarring/pain. | |
| 4. **Controlling Body Temperature** | Temperature 36.5 on admission. No problems | |
| 5. **Eating and Drinking** | Normal diet, appetite good, occasional alcohol, no sugar in drinks. | |
| 6. **Personal Cleansing and Dressing** | No problems with washing and dressing. Takes bath or shower. Has own teeth. | |
| 7. **Communicating** | A pleasant lady who is very open and easy to talk to. Occasional earache causes some hearing loss to L ear. No anxieties. Hopes operation will reduce painful spasms. | |
| 8. **Expressing Sexuality** | Uncomfortable with her clothes 'not hanging right' since segmentectomy. Finds left breast ugly. Husband supportive. Has felt better with silicon prosthesis in bra. | |
| 9. **Sleeping** | Sleeps well but does not breathe too deeply as this is uncomfortable. Has two pillows. 7 – 8 hours total usually. | |
| 10. **Mobilising** | No problems with mobilising, no aids required. | P = Potential deep thrombosis due to immobility post-operatively |
| 11. **Working & Playing** | Badminton coach – full time. Letter writing, knitting, reading. | |
| 12. **Dying** | Very tough lady who tells me she 'does not believe what anyone says until she can see the proof'. Is not therefore afraid of death. Will talk openly as her sister died of cancer recently and there was no communication within the family about her dying/death. Mrs Oakley says she 'will not let that happen again' and 'wants it all in the open'. | |

| NAME: MRS JOANNA MAY OAKLEY. | STANDARD PRE-OPERATIVE CARE PLAN | | | DATES + INITIALS | |
|---|---|---|---|---|---|
| Problem + causes | Goal + goal criteria | Interview | Evaluate | Items discontinued | Nurse recording |
| **Eliminating**<br>Potential incontinence of urine & faeces; due to loss of voluntary muscle control during anaesthetic | Reduce risk of incontinence<br>**Criteria**<br>Bladder and bowels are empty before going to theatre | ● Give suppositories or enema and have evidence of good bowel movement<br>● Ensure bladder is empty before giving premedication | Evening before op.<br>Morning of surgery | | WE 7.6.93<br>WE 8.6.93 |
| **Personal cleansing and dressing**<br>Potential wound infection due to:<br>Bacteria from skin or clothing | Reduce risk of wound infection<br>**Criteria**<br>Skin is intact and smooth after shave. Skin is clean after bath. | ● Shave area appropriate to surgery<br>● Give bath.<br>● Dress in theatre cap and gown<br>● Ensure bed has clean linen and canvas and draw sheet are on bed | Evening before surgery<br>Evening before and morning of operation<br>Morning of surgery | | WE 7.6.93<br>WE 7.6.93 8.6.93<br>WE 8.6.93 |
| **Mobilising**<br>Potential deep vein thrombosis due to immobility | Reduce risk of DVT<br>**Criteria**<br>Appropriate preventive measures taken. | ● Reinforce physiotherapist's teaching of leg and breathing exercises<br>● Unless contra-indicated, encourage mobility during post-operative period | Evening before surgery (Discussed and encouraged) | | WE 7.6.93 |

| NAME: MRS JOANNA MAY OAKLEY. | STANDARD PRE-OPERATIVE CARE PLAN | | | DATES + INITIALS | |
|---|---|---|---|---|---|
| Problem + causes | Goal + goal criteria | Intervention | Evaluate | Items discontinued | Nurse recording |
| **Sleeping**<br>Potential insomnia due to apprehension and strange environment | Refreshing sleep before surgery<br>**Criteria**<br>Observed to sleep for most of the night. States that slept. | ● Ensure quiet<br>● Check comfort of patient before sleep<br>● Give sedative if prescribed/ requested<br>● Milky drink at bedtime if patient so desires | Daily | | Slept well prior to operation<br>WE<br>8.6.93 |
| **Maintaining a safe environment.**<br>Potential injury from:<br>Dentures<br>Contact lenses<br>Spectacles<br>Hearing aid<br>Jewellery<br>Hair clips | No accidential injury due to sharp or breakable personal objects.<br>**Criteria**<br>Patient will understand risk and make sure that personal property is safely kept. | ● Jewellery removed – wedding ring taped.<br>● Remove dentures.<br>● Hearing aid to be removed in anaesthetic room and kept safely in recovery.<br>● Ensure all property stored safely. | Before premedication | | WE<br>8.6.93 |
| Potential wrong patient or wrong operation due to wrong identity or wrong side | Patient will be correctly identified for correct operation<br>**Criteria**<br>Correct patient arrives in theatre for correct operation on correct side. | ● Check name at all handovers<br>● Check with unit nurse.<br>● Check identiband.<br>● Check all case records.<br>● Check correct X-rays. | Morning of surgery | All checked when I collected patient.<br>WE<br>8.6.93 | |

(*continued*)

| Problem | Goal | Nursing action | Time | Evaluation |
|---|---|---|---|---|
| **Communicating**<br>Potential anxiety due to impending operation/ anaesthetic | No excessive anxiety.<br>**Criteria**<br>No signs of undue anxiety.<br>States that feels less anxious. | ● Give opportunity to ask questions about operation.<br>● Give information about what will happen:<br>● during pre-operative preparation in ward<br>● Transfer to theatre<br>● Support during induction of anaesthesia.<br>● Support in recovery room.<br>● Anticipated pattern of post-operative care. incl. IVI drainage tubes.<br>● Pain and availability of analgesia. | At latest – day before surgery. | Discussed during pre-operative visit WE 7.6.93 |
| **Breathing**<br>Potential respiratory problems due to:-<br>Regurgitation/aspiration of gastric contents during induction | Reduce risk of aspiration of gastric contents during induction.<br>**Criteria**<br>Stomach to be empty before induction. | ● Fast for four hours before surgery.<br>● Explain to patient so that patient will cooperate. | Morning of surgery | Discussed during pre-operative visit<br>WE 7.6.93 |

equipment as requested, ensuring illumination of the surgical field, altering the operating light as required and paying meticulous attention to specimens to ensure they are correctly contained, properly labelled and dispatched to the pathological laboratory promptly. Other responsibilities will be the recording of blood loss by weighing swabs, maintaining accurate swab, instrument and needle counts and maintaining accurate documentation of all information pertaining to Mrs Oakley's care so that the recovery and ward teams are fully informed of procedural needs, hazards and complications which could occur and ensure continuity of care.

Mrs Oakley's operation went without complications and she was safely transferred to the recovery room.

A post-operative visit allowed the theatre nurse to evaluate the care given during surgery and to find out how Mrs Oakley was progressing.

Two days post-operatively, Mrs Oakley was in good spirits. She was pleased with the initial results of her reconstruction surgery but had not had an opportunity to see the complete result because of the drains and dressings. Although the wound was still causing her some discomfort she was keen to start her arm exercises as she wanted to return to work as early as possible.

Using Roper's model had enabled the nurse to plan comprehensively to meet any real or potential problems. The activities of living provided a focus for determining care needs and priority. By being involved in her care throughout the peri-operative period the theatre nurse was able to form a meaningful relationship with Mrs Oakley, which helped her cope with the stress of surgery and enabled holistic nursing care.

## Using Orem's model [2] to plan care for Mr Smith who is undergoing surgery for an adrenal tumour

Mr Smith is a 62 year old married gentleman, who originates from Austria. He has lived in this country for the past 30 years and is self-employed running a chauffeur driven car business. He has two grown up children, a son and a daughter, who is married and has recently suffered a miscarriage, which upset Mr Smith.

Recently Mr Smith was involved in a motor cycle accident, sustaining leg injuries and serious injuries to his forehead and nose which required plastic surgery. It was during this admission that a chest X-ray demonstrated a raised right hemidiaphragm. Further investigations revealed an adrenal mass approximately 9 × 11 cm. Initially this was thought to be a haematoma caused by the accident, so he was asked to attend for another appointment two months later.

The mass was still present and although not causing any discomfort, the surgeon advised Mr Smith to undergo surgery to determine the cause.

Mr Smith had a previous history of myocardial infarction and had been a heavy smoker, smoking up to 40 cigarettes a day. Following his accident he had given up smoking and drinking, but found he tired easily and had to retire much earlier, mainly due to the ache in his left leg caused by injuries sustained at the time of his accident.

## Assessment

Mr Smith was assessed during a pre-operative visit by the theatre nurse. He appeared relaxed and was easy to talk to, beginning to chat at once, speaking freely about his earlier life, his family and his business. He was happy to listen to information about his impending surgery, but was not keen to discuss detail.

Orem's model seemed to suit Mr Smith because he was normally able to meet his self-care needs and wanted to take an active part in his care. Following a detailed assessment the nurse was able to formulate a plan of care based on the universal self-care requisites as described by Orem.

Once the operation was completed Mr Smith was transferred to recovery where the nursing role became partially compensatory. The following pages illustrate how the planned care was implemented.

## Evaluation

Mr Smith had an uncomplicated post-operative recovery. During his stay his vital signs remained within normal limits, his oxygen saturation was maintained between 96% and 100% and his respirations between 14–16 breaths per minute and his pain was well controlled. The wound site remained dry and there was minimum drainage from the wound drain. He was able to rest for long periods and when awake communicated well with the nursing staff.

Orem's model worked well for Mr Smith as nursing actions were able to compensate fully in meeting self-care deficits whilst Mr Smith was anaesthetised and became partially compensatory as he returned to consciousness. By the time he was returned to the ward he had regained his self-caring role regarding the ability to maintain oxygenation, maintain balance between rest and sleep and between solitude and social interaction. He was much more in control of maintaining his own safe environment, but would still require further help from nursing staff due to the presence of an intravenous infusion, urinary catheter, wound drain and epidural catheter which would hinder his

## Planning

| Universal self-care requisites | Self-care abilities | Self-care deficits | Potential self-care deficits | Self-care aims and actions | Nursing actions |
|---|---|---|---|---|---|
| Main intake of air. | Normally able to manage respiratory needs without assistance. | No self-care deficits. | The patient may be unable to maintain his own airway (the nurse will compensate wholly). May have difficulty in breathing post-operatively as patient is an ex-smoker. Risk of further respiratory compromise because of incision and drains. Pain on deep breathing may hinder coughing. There is a potential for infection or atelectasis because of immobility and failure to expand lungs fully periodically. | The patient will be able to maintain his own airway. He will be able to breathe without difficulty. Patient will ask for analgesia when needed. Will notify nurse if breathing becomes difficult or painful. Will learn to use splinting technique to breathe/cough. Will learn relaxation techniques during periods of pain. | The nurse will ensure that the patient's airway is patent and will support it to prevent obstruction. Oxygen will be administered until the patient is fully awake and the oxygen saturation and respirations are within normal ranges. Sit patient upright as soon as possible to aid full lung expansion and aid breathing. |
| Maintain intake of fluid. | Able to manage this need. | No self-care deficits. | Patient may be dehydrated due to pre-operative fasting. Patient will have to remain nil by mouth until fully conscious, gag reflex present and not feeling nauseated. Following surgery, there is the potential for fluid loss (including blood). This may affect blood pressure. Therefore the patient will need support in the maintenance of fluid balance. There is also the potential for electrolyte imbalance due to fluid loss or alteration of nutritional status. | Patient will be adequately hydrated intraoperatively and post-operatively until able to drink freely himself. Patient will be able to communicate with nursing staff if nausea is present or if severe thirst develops. Patient will be able to manage own mouth care soon after surgery. | Adequate mouth care given until patient can drink. Intravenous fluids administered as ordered to help maintain hydration. Check intravenous site to ensure that the site is not inflamed or infiltrated. |

| | | | | | |
|---|---|---|---|---|---|
| Maintain intake of food. | Can prepare own meals and has a good understanding of dietary requirements. | No self-care deficits. | Patient will have been fasting for at least six hours pre-operatively and will not be able to resume eating until he is fully conscious, not nauseated and tolerating oral fluids. | Patient will be adequately nourished until he is able to return to taking a normal diet. Patient will be able to alert staff if nausea or vomiting occurs. | Give antiemetic medication as required. Maintain intravenous fluids to provide some nutritional benefits while nil by mouth. Support patient by advising that gut motility often takes several hours to return after surgery. |
| Maintain elimination. | Able to manage this need. | No self-care deficits. | Will be inhibited in his management of his elimination processes by having a urinary catheter in place. Potential for low urinary output due to dehydration. Potential for constipation post-operatively due to immobility, reduction in dietary intake dehydration or morphine based analgesia. Potential for discomfort from catheter due to too much tension being placed on same or feeling of abdominal discomfort which may be due to a kink or blockage of the tubing. | For Mr Smith to return to normal elimination processes as soon as possible and without any complication. To explain to the patient the importance of reporting difficulties he may experience, e.g. discomfort or a feeling of urgency to void. To notify staff if flatulence occurs. | To ensure that there are no kinks or blockage in the tubing. To ensure that there is an adequate urinary output every hour (30mls/hour). To observe the urine for colour and consistency. To explain to the patient that he has a catheter in situ and keep reminding him as he is likely to forget. |

| Universal self-care requisites | Self-care abilities | Self-care deficits | Potential self-care deficits | Self-care aims and actions | Nursing actions |
| --- | --- | --- | --- | --- | --- |
| Balance activity and rest. | Has been able to participate in all his usual activities, for example walking his dog. | He has required much more resting time following his accident due to the ache in his left leg. He has many a restless night because of this. | Patient will probably be on bedrest for the first 24 hours with the potential risk of DVT or chest infection. Pain may also potentially restrict mobility as well as cause restlessness. Regular vital signs may interrupt the patient's rest. There is also the potential problem of being in an unfamiliar environment with noise and light preventing undisturbed rest. Activity may also be restricted due to intravenous therapy and drains. | To ensure that the patient is as pain free as possible, ensure maximum rest periods. For Mr Smith to return to normal mobility as soon as possible. To prevent the complications of bedrest. Patient will understand or anticipate the need for assistance when first mobilising. | Ensure that patient is as comfortable as possible by assessing pain level and give analgesia as required. |
| Balance solitude and social interaction. | Maintains close relationships with his family and friends, but enjoys time by himself. | Had been speaking to the other patients on the ward, but then settled down to reading his book. | Tiredness may be exacerbated by surgery and the use of analgesia post-operatively. Potential to become slightly disorientated by the combination of drugs and the strange environment. May become intolerant of nursing interventions such as regular vital signs and checking wound site and drains. | For Mr Smith to be able to rest when desired, and to be able to feel relaxed about asking questions and communicating with the nursing staff. | Orientate the patient to his surroundings and the time as soon as he is awake. Reassure him and explain all the procedures that are carried out. Encourage him to ask questions. Allow patient time to rest undisturbed. |

| | | | | | |
|---|---|---|---|---|---|
| Prevent hazards to life, well-being and functioning. | Intellectually and physically able to prevent hazards to life if aware of them. | Patient owns his own company which leaves him with stress management difficulties and long working hours. | Mr Smith will be unconscious or sedated for a time in recovery and will not be able to protect himself or avoid injuries caused by uncoordinated movements, drowsiness or restlessness. Following anaesthetic agents and analgesia, the patient may not be able to maintain his own airway and may need assistance. He cannot control what medication is given to him nor can he maintain his blood pressure or temperature within normal limits. | Mr Smith will be able to maintain his own airway and manage his own safety as soon as possible after surgery. (Nurse will compensate wholly until then.) | Ensure that the patient is lying on his side and that his airway is supported until conscious. Reassure to alleviate anxiety and stress. Ensure that as the patient is waking he does not injure himself by hitting his limbs on equipment or furniture. Ensure that patient is fully responsive and coherent before attending to charts, etc. |
| Promote normality, develop and maintain a realistic self-concept. | An intelligent person who communicates his concerns and problems well. Appears to have a realistic self-concept. Realises that he needs to have this operation to find out the origin of the mass. | Appears not to have any obvious self-care problems related to self-concept. | Unsure of the impact of surgery. Patient may become stressed by being in a strange environment and by the disruption to his daily routine. Potential to be disorientated and anxious on waking from anaesthesia. | To ensure that the patient's return to normality is uncomplicated. When awake to feel in control of himself again and relaxed in the care of the nursing team. Verbalise concerns about surgery. Continue to have a realistic self-concept. | Reassure patient and encourage him to ask questions. Orientate patient to time and place and continue to reinforce this as patient may be forgetful following sedation. |

| **Developmental self-care requisites** | **Self-care abilities** | **Self-care deficits** | **Potential self-care deficits** | **Self-care aims and actions** | **Nursing actions** |
|---|---|---|---|---|---|
| Maintain lifestyle that promotes maturation. | Mr Smith takes great pride in his company and enjoys his work. He is a family man and they are very closely knit. | Mr Smith expressed concerns about the length of time that he would need to be away from his work and the possible effects this may have. | Mr Smith may believe that following surgery his life will be back to normal, but there is the possibility that the mass may be malignant and he may need further treatment. He does not mention this. | Patient will be able to discuss his professional and personal development following surgery. | Be supportive of the patient. Allow the patient the opportunity to talk about any possible changes in his life. |
| **Health care deviation self-care requisites** | **Self-care abilities** | **Self-care deficits** | **Potential self-care deficits** | **Self-care aims and actions** | **Nursing actions** |
| Be aware of and attend to pathological conditions and side effects of medical care. | Is aware that there is a mass present and that a specimen needs to be sent to histology to determine its origin. | Not aware of the complications of surgery. | Potential for Mr Smith to be unaware of the possible unpleasant side effects. Mr Smith will need education about this. Potential for Mr Smith to require further treatment such as radiotherapy if the mass is malignant. Patient may not be expecting this. | That Mr Smith will have a good understanding of his operation and be aware that unpleasant side effects such as nausea and pain are likely to occur. To ensure that Mr Smith is aware that he must alert nursing staff if he is uncomfortable, is feeling nauseated or is worried generally. | Ensure that the patient is informed of all treatments given and reasons for same. Explain to the patient that certain side effects of his surgery are normal and reassure him. |

**Implementation of care plan**

1. *Self-care deficits in the maintenance of sufficient intake of air*

Mr Smith's bed space was checked before his arrival in recovery to ensure that the oxygen and suction were working, that a kidney dish was nearby, a catheter stand and a drip pole and the relevant paper work present. Mr Smith arrived in recovery at 1630 hours. He was conscious and self-ventilating. His airway was patent, his cough and swallow reflexes were present and there was no laryngospasm. His colour was good. He was commenced on oxygen 40% via a face mask. His respirations were 16 per minute on arrival and were maintained between 14 and 22 per minute during his stay in recovery. They were recorded every 15 minutes for the first two hours, then half hourly for one hour, then hourly. His respiratory depth and his colour were also recorded. His oxygen saturations were measured using a pulse oximeter. Recordings varied from 96% on arrival up to 100% when settled. Mr Smith arrived in recovery in the left lateral position, supported by pillows. He found this comfortable and was reluctant to be sat upright for the first hour or so, as he was afraid that it would aggravate what pain he already had. He was happy to be sat upright at 1815 hours and felt quite comfortable in this position as the epidural had had time to take effect and his pain was much less. Once Mr Smith was less sleepy, he was encouraged to cough and deep breathe regularly and to continue to do so when he returned to the ward. He was also encouraged to expectorate any secretions present. His oxygen was discontinued at 1900 hours. Mr Smith's respiratory status was very satisfactory on his return to the ward. His respirations were 20 at the time, of good depth, his colour good and his final oxygen saturation was 99%.

2. *Self-care deficits in maintaining sufficient intake of water*

Mr Smith arrived in recovery with a litre of dextrose saline in progress to infuse over eight hours, then to be followed by a litre of normal saline over ten hours. He did not require a blood transfusion during the operation. The intravenous site was checked regularly for redness and infiltration which did not occur. He also had an arterial line in situ which had been used for monitoring in theatre.

It was now capped off and was to be removed a few hours later if there were no post-operative complications as ordered by the anaesthetist. Mr Smith was very dry post-operatively and was given regular mouthwashes. He was advised that he was not to have any oral fluids until he felt better able to tolerate same and to avoid vomiting and therefore strain on his wound. He was told that he could have an injection for nausea, he was bordered for stemetil 12.5 mg 4–6 hourly, but he did not require this. All fluids administered to Mr Smith were recorded on a fluid balance chart, along with his output.

3. *Self-care deficit in maintaining sufficient intake of food*

Mr Smith had received 1 ml of intravenous droperidol in theatre and did not require any further antiemetic in recovery. He was advised that on feeling more alert and able to tolerate substances by mouth, he should begin with sips of water followed by clear fluids and then slowly progress to a light diet. He was reassured that his intravenous fluids would sustain him adequately until then. Mr Smith did begin taking sips of water the following day and slowly progressed to a light diet, although he felt that he did not have much of an appetite for the first few post-operative days.

4. *Self-care deficits associated with elimination*

Mr Smith had a urinary catheter in situ post-operatively. This was secured safely to his leg to prevent traction. This was explained to him initially and this information reinforced at different stages as Mr Smith was quite sleepy to begin with and was likely to forget this. He was asked to inform staff if any discomfort or traction was felt from the catheter. This did not pose a problem. He was on hourly urinary measurements and these remained above 30 ml an hour. His output was accurately recorded and observation on colour and consistency of urine carried out. Mr Smith also had one redivac in situ and this was also explained to him and its hourly measurements recorded. There was minimal drainage from same. It was also secured safely to the patient. Mr Smith was shivering on arrival in recovery and his central temperature was 35.6°C. A space blanket was applied and Mr Smith slowly warmed up to 36.7°C before returning to the ward.

5. *Self-care deficit in maintaining a balance between rest and activity*

Mr Smith had an epidural sited in the anaesthetic room pre-operatively. He had a stat dose of diamorphine 5 mg given through this before he left theatre. He had minimal pain on arrival in recovery. When Mr Smith was settled into recovery, a diamorphine infusion of 15 mg in 60 ml of normal saline was set up and commenced at 0.25 mg an hour. The prescribed dosage was 1–5 ml an hour. Mr Smith was maintained on 0.25 mg an hour during his stay in recovery. This allowed him to rest sufficiently. When Mr Smith was more alert, the importance of passive exercises and deep breathing was explained. He was wearing a pair of TEDs stockings which had been applied pre-operatively and Mr Smith was reminded of the purpose of these and that they would remain in situ until full mobility was achieved. The frequency of vital signs and the noise and lighting of the recovery room did not appear to disturb Mr Smith. He commented in the recovery room that he had asked family members and friends not to visit him the evening of his operation and I felt that this allowed him to rest well, as he was not anticipating any visit or the need to converse with people.

6. *Self-care deficits in maintaining the balance between solitude and social interaction*

When Mr Smith arrived in recovery, he recognised me immediately and said that he was glad to see me. He was orientated to his surroundings and to time. It was reinforced again that his operation was complete and that everything was going to plan. The presence of a drip, catheter, drain, oxygen and pulse oximeter was explained. All procedures were explained to Mr Smith and he was reassured regularly. He was advised to rest as much as possible, but to alert staff if he was uncomfortable or worried in any way. He was very chatty initially, which I felt was partly due to relief that his operation was complete. He then settled and slept intermittently.

7. *Self-care deficits in the prevention of hazards to human life*

Mr Smith was slightly restless and shivering on arrival in recovery and needed reassurance and close observation to prevent him from injuring himself from impacts with pieces of equipment and from pulling on his drip, catheter and drain. He settled down shortly afterwards following explanation on what was happening and on being orientated to his surroundings.

His airway was fully patent and did not require any support, although he required oxygen to maintain his oxygen saturations within normal limits until fully awake and sitting upright.

Mr Smith's vital signs were recorded 1/4 hourly initially to detect any problems with blood pressure or heart rate. Patients with hyperfunction of the adrenal cortises frequently experience hypertension.

Mr Smith has a non-functioning right adrenal gland prior to surgery, so this was not a problem for him. His wound and Redivac were observed frequently in case haemorrhaging occurred.

His fluid intake and output were monitored to prevent under or overloading him and to ensure that he was voiding satisfactorily. Mr Smith's temperature was low on arrival in recovery. A space blanket was applied to help to rewarm him and to perfuse his tissues and help prevent hypothermia.

8. *Self-care deficits in the promotion of the human desire to be normal and to develop and maintain a realistic self-concept.*

   Mr Smith recognised me straight away and was very relieved that his operation was complete. He was alert but slightly disorientated when he first arrived in recovery. He was quickly orientated and reassured and the presence of the various drips and tubes was explained to him. He was encouraged to ask questions and was reassured that a nurse would be with him at all times.

9. *Self-care deficits in maintaining a lifestyle that promotes maturation*

   Mr Smith enquired how his operation had gone and whether the tumour was now gone. He also enquired about how long it would be before he could move about freely again. Truthful responses to all of his questions were forthcoming, as far as current information allowed.

10. *Self-care deficit in the ability to be aware of and to attend to pathological conditions and side effects of medical care*

    It was explained to Mr Smith that his incision site was likely to cause pain on breathing but that he had an epidural in situ which could be increased in dosage if he needed this. He was also informed of the potential for the feeling of nausea, but again reassured that he could have medication to counteract this. Finally, Mr Smith was informed that he would feel tired, lacking in energy and probably lose his appetite for the first few days, but that these side effects of surgery would pass and were quite normal.

progress as he began to mobilise. By encouraging the patient to do as much for himself as possible, Mr Smith was empowered to take control which helped to promote his recovery and well-being. These two care studies demonstrate how nursing care can be enhanced by use of a theoretical framework to guide the process of nursing. The models chosen are probably those you are most familiar with and we hope you can see how they ensure nursing care is systematic, planned to meet individual client needs and holistic, recognising biopsychosocial needs.

*Activity*

Roper's model works very well in most acute care settings and is widely used throughout the United Kingdom, perhaps because it is a British model and therefore is easily understood.

Can you see any weaknesses in the model as used to plan Mrs Oakley's care?

*Activity*

Orem's model is less well known in this country and is perhaps less well used, partly due to the unfamiliar terminology used to describe the underpinning principles, but it does have a lot to offer when planning care for individuals who are essentially independent and have the ability to be self-caring. It places emphasis on client involvement, the nursing role being to assist, encourage and educate.

Try to identify how these principles are demonstrated in Mr Smith's care.

When you have the opportunity, perhaps you will use another model as a framework for assessing and planning nursing care. Ask your clinical supervisor or your educational advisor which model would be appropriate and try it out.

## References

1. Roper, N, Logan, W and Tierney, A (1985) *The Elements of Nursing*, 2nd edn. Churchill Livingstone, Edinburgh.
2. Orem, DE (1991) *Nursing: Concepts of Practice*, 4th edn. McGraw-Hill, New York.

## Further reading

Aggleton, P and Chalmers, H (1986) *Nursing Models and the Nursing Process*. MacMillan Education Ltd, London.

Cavanagh, SJ (1991) *Orem's Model in Action*. MacMillan Press Ltd, London.

Newton, C. (1991) *The Roper-Logan-Tierney Model in Action*. MacMillan Press Ltd, London.

Walsh, M. (1991) *Models in Clinical Nursing: The Way Forward*. Baillière Tindall, London

Wright, SG (1990) *Building and Using a Model of Nursing*. Edward Arnold, London.

# 10 The Role of the Nurse

We hope your experiences in theatre and the suggested exercises have helped you clarify what the nurse's role in theatre is and perhaps before reading further, you would like to jot down your ideas.

We hope you will be able to see that this is not fundamentally different from any other nursing role. Perhaps the nurse requires some extra skills to manage the technical nature of practice but these should not be seen in isolation, as a series of tasks; they are just one part of the holistic role of the nurse, which should be 'to assist the patient . . . in those activities contributing to health, or recovery, or a peaceful death'.[1]

## Role of the theatre nurse

Many writers have questioned the role of the nurse in theatre.[2,3,4] McGee suggests that, in part, this is due to the alien theatre environment and the fact that the theatre nurse may never get to know the patient. We hope that you have been able to see how the theatre nurse can change this image by encompassing the peri-operative role; participating in pre-operative preparation; planning individualised care, which is based on biopsychosocial needs; implementing and evaluating goals, thus fulfilling the UKCC *Code of Conduct* and providing a quality service.[5]

Others[3,6] have demonstrated how easy it is for the theatre nurse to get caught up in the technology of operating theatre work, finding little time to take up the challenge of the peri-operative role, thus becoming a handmaiden to the surgeon rather than an advocate for the patient. In the current climate of cost cutting, it is important that the theatre nurse can justify her position.

Benner[7] has written extensively about nursing practice and she identified seven domains of nursing, These, she suggests, include:

1. a helping role;
2. a teaching/coaching function;
3. a diagnosis and patient monitoring function;

4. effective management of rapidly changing situations;
5. administration and monitoring therapeutic interventions and treatments;
6. monitoring and evaluating quality health care;
7. organisation and work role competences.

The theatre nursing role can encompass all these domains.

We hope you have been able to identify and relate to these functions through the activities we have suggested and, more importantly, by the examples of the nursing staff you have been working with.

Benner also proposed several stages of development from novice to expert in nursing practice, making the distinction between the competent practitioner, who may be able to manage a wide range of clinical situations, and the expert, who can use clinical experience and intuition to see the situation as a whole and provide 'holistic' care.

It may have been difficult for you to separate these roles out, but perhaps you have accompanied a nurse on a pre-operative visit and observed how she has been able to help the patient express and manage anxiety. You may also have been able to provide help and information related to surgery and recovery, thus empowering the patient to take an active role in their care. Part of the purpose of the pre-operative visit is to assist the nurse in gaining information related to the patient's specific needs in theatre, to prepare for and meet these. For example an elderly patient might be at particular risk of inadvertent hypothermia during surgery.[8,9] The theatre nurse's role would be to identify this and plan appropriate strategies to ensure body temperature is maintained within acceptable limits, thus avoiding hazards and complications related to, for example, drug elimination.

We have shown you how nurses can plan systematic care, using an identified framework, to ensure the patient's individual needs are met and continuity of care is assured. The theatre nurse needs to be familiar with a variety of nursing models, as she may be continuing care from widely differing philosophical standpoints and it will be important to understand how initial assessment and goal setting have been identified.

Within the operating department you may find that intraoperative care is 'standardised' as many of the goals of care will be similar. This should not detract from treating the patient as an individual but will ensure all normative needs are met.[10]

The last four domains are probably easier for you to relate to as rapidly changing situations occur frequently and you have, no doubt, observed how the teamwork in theatre ensures these are managed with efficiency and effectiveness. Theatre nurses are in an ideal position to respond to the UKCC *Scope of Professional Practice*,[11] as they actively participate in therapeutic interventions by acting as first assistant to surgeons or anaesthetists. The potential for role expansion in responding to the challenges of surgery is great, and is reflected in the work role competences required.

Melton[12] eloquently describes theatre nurses as:

> professional nurses who have mastered the fine art of pantomime. They speak through the expression of their eyes and give assurance with the touch of a hand. They are endowed with the knowledge of a unit nurse, the mechanical ability of a trained professional, the electrical swiftness of a computer, and the patience of a nun

She elaborates further in stating the theatre nurse is the 'eyes, ears and mouth' and also 'the heart and the hands' of her patient; a psychiatrist, engineer, chemist and microbiologist, teacher, counsellor and educator.

We hope this book has helped you to see that the holistic role of the nurse is greater than the sum of the parts, that it is an essential role to ensure patients receive the care they need during this important and vulnerable stage of their care and that it offers many challenges and rewards.

We hope you have enjoyed your experience and even if this field of nursing is not for you, that you have learned a lot about patient care in the operating theatre, which will help you prepare patients for, and provide, informed post-operative care.

## References


1. Henderson, V (1966) *The Nature of Nursing*. Collier MacMillan, London.
2. Fennell, L (1989) But is it nursing? *B J Theatre Nursing*, Feb, **26** (2) 13–17.
3. Johnson, G (1990) Preop visits: why they don't happen. *Nursing*, **4** (19), 24–27.
4. McGee, P (1992) Theatre nurses face elimination. *B J Nursing*, **1** (11), 535–536.
5. United Kingdom Central Council (1992) *Code of Professional Conduct*. UKCC, London.
6. Baxter, B (1987) Crisis in theatre – shortage of theatre nurses. *N Times*, **83** (40), 63–64.
7. Benner, P (1984) *From Novice to Expert: Excellence and Power in Clinical Nursing Practice*. Addison-Wesley, California.
8. Surkitt-Parr, M (1992) Hypothermia in surgical patients. *Nursing*, **1** (11), 539–545.
9. Fox, J (1993) Chilling facts. *N. Times*, **89** (41), 18–22.

10. West, B (1993) Caring, thc essence of theatre nursing. *Theatre Nursing*, **3** (8) (suppl), 15–26.
11. United Kingdom Central Council (1992) *The Scope of Professional Practice*. UKCC, London.
12. Melton, B (1982) Operating room nurses, who needs them? *NAT News*, September, 12.

## Further reading

Harris, S (1991) The role of the theatre nurse. *Paed Nursing*, Feb **3** (1), 13–19.

Wicker, P (1990) A reassuring presence. *N. Times*, **86** (29), 59–60.

# GLOSSARY

**Accountable** Bound to give account.

**Advocacy** Pleading for, speaking for another. Used in a very specific way to help to define the professional role of the nurse.

**Anaesthetic gases (expired)** The expired lung contents of the anaesthetised or recently anaesthetised patient.

**Anaesthetic room** That room in the operating department where the patient is normally anaesthetised (in the UK) before transfer to the operating theatre itself.

**Analgesia** (Adj) Absence of pain. Usually used to refer to drugs which relieve pain.

**Antisepsis** Word used to describe processes which reduce the number of active micro-organisms, used particularly when unable to carry out full disinfection or *sterilisation*, e.g. skin antisepsis.

**Asepsis** Absence of infection. Aseptic technique describes the technique involving *sterilisation* which is used to prevent wound infection.

**Audit** Formal procedure for measuring standards.

**Autonomy** The right of self-government, having the freedom to act independently.

**Baseline record** A measurement which is meaningless in isolation but which allows comparison of subsequent measurements to be made, e.g. pre-operative record of vital signs.

**Communication** Process of imparting information, consciously or unconsciously.

**Compliance** An action in accordance with a request. (Also used to describe the physical process of yielding to a force, e.g. lung compliance.)

**Consent** Give permission or agree to something.

**COSHH regulations** Regulations to control the use of substances hazardous to health in the workplace.

**Criterion** Principle or standard against which something is judged. (Referenced assessment)

**Culture** Customs, beliefs and values of a particular time, group or civilisation.

**Departmental manager** Person who has the authority to make decisions regarding the acquisition and utilisation of departmental resources.

**Diathermy** Short wave (radio frequency) electricity used to control bleeding and cut tissue during surgery. (Electrosurgery)

**Disinfectant** Substance or method used to destroy active micro-organisms. Will not destroy spores in the normally prescribed time span.

**Empathy** Identifying with the feelings of another.

**Endoscope** Instrument with series of lenses for viewing the inside of body cavities.

**Endosurgery** Surgery carried out under endoscopic visualisation.

**Fume cabinet** Ventilated cabinet for use when handling substances which produce toxic or carcinogenic fumes

**General anaesthetic** An induced state of altered consciousness, analgesia and muscle relaxation.

**Glutaraldehyde** Aldehyde, related to formaldehyde, used in theatres to disinfect instruments which cannot be heat sterilised. Toxic. See *COSHH regulations*.

**Gowning and gloving** Process of washing hands to remove as many micro-organisms as possible before donning sterilised gown and gloves to carry out or assist with surgery.

**HCA** Health Care Assistant. Level 2 NVQs in theatre only.

**Homeostasis** State of equilibrium maintained by physiological processes.

**Humanistic** Descriptive of the study of man in terms of social and psychological make-up.

**Hypovolaemia** Depletion of blood volume, usually by haemorrhage or fluid loss.

**Internalisation** Assimilation of beliefs and values into the personality of an individual.

**Intolerance** Lack of toleration leading to rejection of a substance in a particular situation.

**Laminar flow** Flow of air or liquid along constant (layered) streamlines without turbulence.

**Local anaesthesia** Loss of sensation at a specific site, induced by application or injection of local anaesthetic agents (e.g. Lignocaine).

**Medical diagnosis** Label given to a pathological disorder.

**Medical problem** Problem associated with medical prescribing or treatment.

**Mentor** Experienced and trusted supervisor. Sometimes used with varying meanings in nurse education.

**Minimally invasive surgery** (see *Endosurgery*) Surgery avoiding major incisions to allow access to the operating site, tending to enable rapid recovery and early discharge.

**Nursing problem** Problem requiring nursing intervention according to nursing diagnosis.

**NVQ** National Vocational Qualification.

**ODA** Operating Department Assistant, sometimes known as theatre technician or medical technical officer.

**ODP** The Operating Department Practitioner is the new theatre person who has completed an NVQ training.

**OEL** Occupational Exposure Level. Relates to the measurement of exposure levels to substances hazardous to health.

**Operating department** The anaesthetic room, operating theatre and recovery area are the three main areas of the operating department. There is sometimes a patient reception area as well.

**Operative procedure** Blanket term to cover all procedures carried out in the operating department and including non-invasive, diagnostic and therapeutic procedures.

**Particle count** Method of measuring the number of particles the same size as micro-organisms to allow an estimate of the cleanliness of the air in an operating theatre.

**Pathologist** One who studies disease processes, especially infections.

**PCA** Patient-controlled analgesia usually an infusion pump controlled by the patient.

**Peri-operative period** That period before, during and after surgery when peri-operative nursing care is carried out and may even start in the outpatient department. This is not a fixed time. During day care this may be the only nursing care given but, for inpatients, pre- and post-operative care will blend into the care given by other groups of nurses.

**Peristalsis** Natural wavelike motion of the gastrointestinal tract which moves contents from mouth to anus.

**Philosophy** Ideas, beliefs, knowledge and perceptions which underlie behaviour.

**Post-operative care** Immediately after an anaesthetic the patient receives one to one nursing care until able to guard his own airway. The post-operative, or recovery, period continues until the patient has recovered from the more disabling effects of the anaesthetic.

**Pre-operative care** Nursing care carried out immediately before surgery. It includes the assessment stage of the peri-operative nursing process.

**Pump technician** An enhanced role of ODAs in which they assist to bypass the heart during open heart surgery.

**Role** A function fulfilled by an individual for a period of time in order to achieve an aim.

**Scavenger system** An exhaust system which contains and takes the patient's expired gases out of the operating theatre and protects the staff from high exposure levels. Gases may include isoflurane, enflurane, halothane or nitrous oxide.

**Scientific** Pertaining to knowledge gained by experimentation and systematically tested.

**Scrubbing** The use of chemical disinfection agents to perform a surgical hand washing technique, the aim being to reduce the resident skin microbes to the lowest possible level. See also *Antisepsis*.

**Scrub team** The surgeon and his assistants who have scrubbed, gowned and gloved to carry out an operative procedure.

**Skin preparation** Term used to describe the skin cleansing process preceding an operation. See also *Antisepsis*.

**Sterile field** Area round the operative site once it has been covered by sterile drapes, which includes the instrument trolley and all of the team who are scrubbed, gowned and gloved.

**Sterilisation** Destruction of all microbes, including spores.

**Suture** A stitch. Suture material includes natural and manmade fibres. When used as a tie rather than a stitch, this is known as a ligature.

**Symbiotic** Cooperation of individuals for mutual gain. Of mutual benefit.

**Team leader** May be a leader of a team of nurses or a leader of a multidisciplinary team.

**Universal precautions** Internationally recognised precautions taken to protect both patients and staff when exposed to blood and body fluids. Based on the premise that all body fluids are potentially infectious. The need for special precautions is assessed against the risk in the situation, not by patient status.

**Value system** Means by which an individual places a value upon something, usually culturally and socially defined.

**Ventilation system** The system by which air is continually changed to maintain clean air in the operating environment. Air is filtered, monitored and temperature and humidity controlled.

# Index